The Ca[...]m
And w[...]

Using Hypnotherapy, Spiritualism
And Conventional Treatments
To Help You Feel Stronger

Louise Evans

Manor House

Cancer Conundrum / Louise Evans

Library and Archives Canada Cataloguing in Publication

Evans, Louise, 1952-, author
    The cancer conundrum : and ways of dealing with it : using hypnotherapy, spiritualism and conventional treatments to help you feel stronger / Louise Evans.

Includes bibliographical references.
ISBN 978-1-988058-43-6 (softcover).-

-ISBN 978-1-988058-44-3 (hardcover)

    1. Cancer--Alternative treatment. 2. Cancer--Treatment. 3. Hypnotism--Therapeutic use. 4. Spiritual healing and spiritualism.
I. Title.

RC271.A62E94 2018   616.99'406   C2018-906175-8

First Edition.
Cover Design-layout / Interior- layout: Michael Davie
144 pages. All rights reserved.
Published Oct. 21, 2018
Manor House Publishing Inc.
452 Cottingham Crescent, Ancaster, ON, L9G 3V6
www.manor-house.biz   (905) 648-2193

Please Note: Author is donating a portion of her net proceeds to the BC Cancer Agency for cancer research.

"This project has been made possible [in part] by the Government of Canada. « *Ce projet a été rendu possible [en partie] grâce au gouvernement du Canada.*"

Funded by the Government of Canada
Financé par le gouvernement du Canada | Canada

Cancer Conundrum / Louise Evans

For my husband Roy and our children
Tara, Heidi, David and Kayla.

Acknowledgements:

I'd like to thank my husband Roy and our children, Tara, Heidi, David and Kayla for all their love and support during my encounter with cancer. I also extend my appreciation to the BC Cancer Agency and doctors and nurses who helped me. Without you I would not have survived. Special thanks to Theresa Davies, Robin Goldfarb, Laurie McGrath and Shirle Schweers, wonderful friends who were there for me in my darkest hour. To all my clients particularly the cancer group I'm very grateful for your invaluable input to this book. Thanks also to the Canadian Society of Clinical Hypnosis (BC Division) for piquing my interest in hypnotherapy and being such excellent teachers. Finally to Manor House I extend my gratitude for editing and publishing this book. To all of you I am forever indebted. The complementary therapies I offer in this book are a mixture of old and new techniques. I've made an effort to be original in my hypnotherapy scripts, but techniques: The Coin Drop (pioneered by Alexander A. Levitan, M.D.), Progressive Muscle Relaxation (created by Edmund Jacobson), Arm Levitation (developed by Milton Erickson) and Eye Fixation (founded by James Braid) are traditional ways of entering trance and have been in use for years. Recognized therapeutic techniques I use in my practice are included in the inductions and some of the ideas come from great writers, who have inspired me over the years, including: Ronald A. Havens, PhD., D. Corydon Hammond, Ph.D., Catherine Walters, M.A., M.S.W. Roger P. Allen Dp Hyp PsyV, George Gafner, CISW, Sonja Benson, Ph.D., and Yvonne M.Dolan.

Disclaimer

Readers of this book should first consult a medical professional as treatments may have an element of risk, even hypnotherapy, which may sometimes result in dizziness, tiredness, anxiety, headaches or false memories. Those suffering from extreme depression, anxiety or other forms of mental illness, should obtain professional help before using any treatments. Do your research prior to embarking on any treatment. Author and publisher are not responsible for any loss, claim or harm arising from the use or misuse of the content herein.

Foreword

Geographically my story begins in the Shetland Islands many years ago and since then I've traveled thousands of miles not only on a world map but emotionally as well.

Life takes so many twists and turns, we are up and we are down, it can be a veritable roller coaster.

Reeling from a cancer diagnosis creates a sinking feeling and there are definite lows but if we are able to survive, the highs that follow can be greater than the lows.

Cancer taught me to slow down and appreciate what I had. It made it very clear that life is a gift and should not be taken for granted. Nearly dying prompted me to fully live.

I remember the period of time between discovering the lump and finding out that it was malignant. Time passed slowly and I fervently prayed and pleaded with God to make that lump benign.

Once my worst fears were realized however and the cancer confirmed I changed my request and asked for survival. Luckily he answered that prayer!

Through the darkest times, listening to my hypnotherapy recordings and journaling helped a great deal, and what started out as a diary of sorts, evolved into much more, culminating in this book.

As you're about to read, the spiritual message I received from my mother, through my channeling friend Robin, changed my whole perspective. To hear from a loved one on the other side that I would survive gave me hope.

Suddenly I believed life would go on and I began to look for the good things the disease had afforded me. There was a shift – my entire thought process changed.

Mindset is crucial particularly when we're unwell. Though I know it may be extremely difficult, depending on one's circumstances, but it is healing to find positivity in the most dire situation and hypnotherapy can help you to do that.

This book is by no means academic however it is important for the reader to be aware that research on the effectiveness of hypnotherapy is ongoing.

Recent studies show that hypnotherapy **appears to improve** mental and physical health in cancer patients (Sharma, 2017) and that when hypnotherapy sessions are given to patients with breast cancer who are undergoing chemotherapy the cognitive and social functioning of these patients is improved. In essence, **this suggests** they have a better quality of life during treatment (Sanchez, 2017)

Research also shows that hypnosis can provide anxiety relief in cancer patients (Chen, Lui, & Chen, 2017) and increase self esteem and optimism (Jaime-Bernal, 2017). In addition it reduces the frequency and severity of hot flashes in breast cancer survivors (Dizon, 2013) and reduces and manages pain in cancer patients (Elkins, Johnson, & Fisher, 2012). Readers should always first obtain professional medical advice before starting any treatment of any kind.

As our body of knowledge and our expertise grows it seems likely that hypnotherapy will become an adjunct in the treatment of cancer.

This book allows me to share therapeutic tools I used during and after treatment, such as prayer, meditation, hypnotherapy, enjoying the outdoors and appreciating nature, spending time with loved ones and taking alone time for contemplation.

These are just some of the ways I coped with cancer. All helped greatly and I was also able to use my counseling knowledge and apply it.

The Gestalt technique of conversing with body parts was beneficial as was desensitization with regards to accepting my altered breast and temporary baldness. Both provided relief.

Exercise became a strong focus and I now attend Treloar Physiotherapy Clinic in Vancouver because they have cancer recovery exercises with trained therapists.

In addition to exercising frequently I still try to eat a healthy balanced diet with plenty of fruit and vegetables.

Cancer made me think carefully about how I wanted to spend my remaining time, and it spurred me into doing things I had always wanted to do but never got round to.

As you'll read, my visit to John of God, the channeling medium and healer in Brazil, was on my bucket list and it turned out to be life changing and truly a miracle.

I hope that on reading my book you will explore hypnotherapy and the other treatments that helped me and may help you as well to become mentally and physically stronger and capable of truly enjoying life.

You'll also read the inspiring stories of my fellow cancer patients and perhaps find solace and comfort as they did in embracing unconventional treatments that offer benefits.

It's time to reprioritize our lives, focus on what is truly important to us and enjoy life to the fullest.

We are survivors.

- Louise Evans

Table of Contents:

Acknowledgements / Disclaimer   4

Foreword   5

1: The Diagnosis   9

2: Just Be Positive   17

3: Treatment   27

4. Anxiety and Depression   37

5: John of God   42

6: Going Forward   51

7: Inductions for Fear and Anxiety   65

8: Inductions During Treatment   79

9: Inductions for Healing   97

10: Inductions to Cope with Depression   113

11: Interlives   127

12: Conclusion   138

About the Author   143

References   144

1: The Diagnosis

My story begins 40 years ago in a small hospital in the Shetland Islands, off the north coast of Scotland.

A screen is pulled up around a hospital bed and behind it a small group of people huddle around one of the patients. That patient is me, a 21 year old female with a compressed vertebra resulting from a car accident.

The screen afforded some privacy and my visitors were heartily enjoying themselves smoking, drinking and socializing. No doubt, all that could be seen by the other patients in the ward were the occasional puffs of smoke as they wafted gently into the air.

Granted we were rather noisy but the nurses and other patients were lenient. In those days Shetlanders (the younger generation, at least) carried a bottle of whisky in their inside pockets and being generous and kind hearted they always offered to share it with their friends, so bottles were passed around from one thirsty mouth to another. Needless to say I declined but regardless we were having fun and my mind was not focused on my injuries.

When visiting hour ended the screens were taken away and I could again see the other patients.

A woman in her 40s lay in the bed opposite me and I noticed she never had any visitors. Sadly, the nurse told me that she had been diagnosed with breast cancer and had just had a mastectomy. I remember thinking at the time, how awful and making a mental note to talk to her later but before I had a chance she was discharged...

... Fast forward 41 years and I am now married and living in Canada. My husband and I have 4 adult children, 2 of whom live with us while the other two live close by. Our lives are pleasantly predictable, we work hard, play when we can and live busy, productive lives.

On the surface, everything appears to be fine. My health has been good apart from the fact that for over 10 years I have had a mysterious, heavy, numbness in my right arm and leg, which generally lasts a day or two every month. Since testing has been unable to identify a cause my doctor believes the symptoms are due to migraines.

During Spring Break in 2014 the numbness returned, only this time it persisted for 12 days forcing me to go to the doctor for a checkup, and, lo and behold, much to everyone's surprise I ended up with a diagnosis of breast cancer, Stage three, Grade three! Memories of the woman in Shetland came flooding back.

My family has always believed in psychics because my mother and her parents received accurate readings over the years from a woman whom they trusted. My grandmother herself was somewhat gifted and read the tealeaves for fun. As a result I was brought up to believe that some people have special gifts and that there is a spiritual realm.

 We were also sent to church on a regular basis and although I continue to believe in God I no longer adhere to one specific religion. The God I believe in loves everybody regardless of race or creed.

It's true that terrible things happen every day to good people-and it's hard to understand why. I believe that we have lessons to learn and agree before our birth to the life we are offered in order to transcend to higher levels on the other side.

I also believe in the possibility of reincarnation, so if we are poor and face health challenges now, perhaps we were rich and healthy in a previous life. That is the only way I can make sense of it.

Of course there are times when I'm shrouded in doubt and think that there's probably nothing after death. Then, I console myself with the thought that before my birth I knew nothing so most likely after death I will know nothing. Most of the time however I feel hopeful that God and an afterlife exist...

...Returning to Shetland once more and rewinding back 41 years my story continues. At that time a group of us, twenty in total, had just graduated from Stirling University in Scotland and had decided to spend one last summer together before venturing out into the world.

One of the boys was from Shetland and he helped us get work in the fish factory and find accommodation so that we could all have fun together. No doubt we smelled terrible but our saving grace was the fact that we smelled terrible en masse!

That summer we met Frank Watt, an amazing clairvoyant who was able to see a person's past, present and future. He worked at the fish factory so my friend Helen and I went to have our fortunes read and we wrote down everything he told us in our travel diaries. Forty-two years later I still have a record of his predictions, about 85% of which proved to be accurate. His gift was exceptional, so good in fact that Bette Davis (the movie star) heard about him and asked for a reading. Frank obliged and sent her a letter outlining his predictions and apparently she was delighted.

Amongst other things Frank told me that I would live a long and healthy life until near the end and I believed him. Now long to me meant living well into my 80s or 90s and since the majority of his predictions had turned out to be remarkably accurate, I sailed through life without a backward glance. I worked hard and played hard, had four great children, possessed endless energy and took it all for granted because Frank had told me it would be so ...

... Now back to the present day: I realize a long life is a subjective matter and since Frank was only 21 when he read to us, it's possible that 62 years (the age at which I received my cancer diagnosis) seemed like a long life to him. I on the other hand was stunned, shocked, in total disbelief. How can you feel so healthy, be so active and suddenly find you have cancer?!!

The mysterious, tired, numb feeling I had experienced for over a decade was inconvenient but really just a trifling as it rarely bothered me and when it did the discomfort only lasted for a short time.

Then, over Spring Break it became more persistent going on for days, forcing me to go to the doctor. Initially my MD wasn't sure what was happening but she was going away for a week and asked me to book a complete checkup upon her return.

Ironically, on the morning of the appointment, I woke up feeling extremely anxious (perhaps on a deeper level, some part of me knew what was to come) but still I was puzzled by my emotions.

As I lay on the examination table I never anticipated the doctor's words as she examined my breasts.

"There's a lump," her voice was grave but controlled and from the tone I knew the lump was fairly large. "Do you do breast self exams?" she asked.

"No". I replied. There were two reasons for this, one I didn't like the feel of my breasts and two, I was afraid I might find something.

"How about mammograms?" she asked.

"No, not any more, I went years ago and it was very uncomfortable. Anyway I didn't think I would ever get breast cancer because none of the females in my family had it".

"I see," she said. "Well I checked you last year and there was nothing obvious then, but let's get a mammogram and ultrasound done right away to see what's happening."

I was stunned and literally shaking when I went back into the waiting room, then out of the doctor's office and into the radiology department.

My husband and I were both distraught on hearing the news: The results of their findings: "It looks highly suspicious for cancer." This was later confirmed with a core biopsy and a lumpectomy. I had Stage 3 Grade 3 breast cancer in my right breast.

The speed at which these events started happening was phenomenal, one moment I was leading an ordinary life and feeling normal and the next, all hell broke loose. It's hard to get your head around it.

During the procedures that followed, the kindness of the people in the health profession profoundly touched me. Of course the vast majority of us are respectful and competent in our place of work, as are the people in the labs and hospitals but there are a few who go above and beyond. To those people I say a big, "Thank you. What you do has a lasting impact."

The doctor who performed my core biopsy let me know what to expect. He said: "I will count to three and then you will hear the click of the machine."

I nodded and tensed my body waiting for the ominous sound. He said: "One, two, three..." and as the machine clicked he then added an extra "Ouch!" for effect.

Actually, there was no pain and somehow that 'ouch' made everything technical so much more human, so much more compassionate. It was as if he was responding to the frightened child in me. My fear dissipated and I was able to see some humor in the situation.

Waiting to hear if the tumor was cancerous was one of the worst times in my life. I was petrified, hoping and praying that it would prove benign.

I remember that first appointment with the surgeon, sitting in the waiting room with my husband and children by my side.

All of us were afraid to breathe.

My family and I experienced a high level of stress that day waiting for the news. After spending what seemed like an eternity in the reception area (my doctor was delayed at the hospital) the surgeon just spoke about the upcoming surgery and informed us that the biopsy results had not yet reached him.

In a way there was a positive slant to this, it was almost like a dress rehearsal because although we stopped holding our breath and relaxed for a while the next visit was not as stressful even though the news was chilling.

Having previously believed that I was healthy and would live to reach my 80s or even my 90s (erroneously assumed by me through misinterpreting Frank's predictions) it came as a tremendous shock to learn that the lump in my breast was Stage 3 cancer.

Panic set in and I didn't know what to do. The doctor spoke about surgery, chemotherapy and radiation, in a matter of fact way since those are the conventional methods of treatment and I tried to listen but inside my thoughts were racing. Should I follow his advice or try a different route? It was a real dilemma, a true conundrum.

I moved through shock, disbelief, terror, denial, and ultimately acceptance and my family suffered with me. It was a painful, frightening time and terror and disbelief were my constant companions. In the end I decided to follow conventional treatments initially and supplement these with complementary therapies.

Once the decision had been made, things happened quickly and the wheels were set in motion.

Numerous statements were bandied about by my surgeon, oncologist, and nurses. "We will remove the tumor from your breast and the lymph nodes." "You will lose your hair but it's only temporary." "You may have a portocath put in your chest."

Dumbfounded, I nodded in agreement. This was so unreal, as though it wasn't really happening to me... it was as if I was a character in a movie, a really scary movie.

"A great read! As a retired hypnotherapist-counsellor I found it an easy to follow interesting read... full of helpful suggestions for anyone with cancer. Thank you Louise for ... such a well presented, insightful and informative book."

- **Emi Kordyback,** MA, hypnotherapist, former registered clinical counselor,

2: Just Be Positive

After receiving a diagnosis of cancer, everyone told me: "Just be positive!" The doctors, nurses, oncologist, family and friends all said this in a well-meaning way. But how could I be positive when faced with a potentially fatal disease? In fact, it became quite irritating and I wanted to scream out: *Shut up, leave me alone and see how you would feel if you were me – how the hell can I be positive?* Images of death and suffering seemed more realistic than putting on a fake Pollyanna smile.

Like a drowning man, I floundered and needed something to hang on to, some shred of hope and comfort which fortunately came to me from an unusual source. One of my closest friends, Robin, is an intuitive healer and channeler and while meditating she was contacted by my deceased mother and given the following message, which she promptly relayed:

'Your mother says you need to control your thoughts. You need to stop jumping so far ahead with crazy ideas and really be in the moment because this is such a big lesson you're going through. It's one of the biggest challenges of your life and you will meet amazing people and go through a lot of hard stuff. She says you have an incredible sense of humor and this will save you. You're so compassionate and that will also lead you on to many other paths when you get through this challenge, get beyond this challenge…

Your life will go in many directions you hadn't planned on and be very strong in other areas that you want to focus on. Your path will become so much more solidified. You don't realize how much you give to this world and through this challenge you will give even more in ways you never imagined. This disease is a true gift. You bring comfort to so many and now you must trust that many will bring comfort to you'. My mother asked Robin to share this message with me and to ask me to, "Please trust."

Her words gave me great hope, in fact they may have saved my life because my mother said *I would survive* and that I had a future. Relief flooded through me. Now whether or not the message was real, some would argue otherwise, belief is the cornerstone of life and the content was a reframe, which completely changed my perspective.

It's thanks to my mother, and my friend Robin, that I am writing this book, which I believe will help me through my treatments and hopefully help some of you who have been diagnosed with this disease. Instead of dwelling on the pain, nausea and fear of chemotherapy, radiation and surgery let's utilize resources. Let's use assets, which will help us travel through these uncharted waters with courage, hope, determination, and perhaps a sprinkling of humor.

Being a counselor and hypnotherapist and spiritual in nature, I decided to utilize all of my assets in order to empower myself and I urge you the reader to do the same. For me these included prayer, meditation, hypnotherapy, adequate sleep, gentle exercise, a healthy balanced diet with lots of fruit and vegetables and quality time with family and friends.

The way to good health was – and is – absolutely clear: Body, mind and soul have to work together in harmony.

Now, everyone's circumstances are unique and you may have different spiritual/religious beliefs, mobility problems, perhaps you have strict dietary guidelines and your family and friends are not nearby, so some of these assets are inaccessible.

However if you truly want to empower yourself then meditation and hypnotherapy are tools that you can use.

Sadly, hypnotherapy has been given a bad rap. Hollywood sensationalizes it and portrays the false idea of being controlled by the therapist and doing things that are unprincipled or even criminal. Stage hypnotists make it look like we are all going to quack like ducks or act in an idiotic fashion when hypnotized. This is just not so. Admittedly, hypnotherapy may have side effects (tiredness, anxiety, headaches, dizziness or production of false memories) but these are extremely rare. However, it's wise to check with your medical practitioner before using it.

The way I use hypnosis makes clients feel good, it helps us use the power of the subconscious mind for healing, and it is relaxing and easy to use. Also and most importantly when we are at our weakest and lying in bed unable to do anything else we can use hypnosis. We can listen to the words and accelerate our healing. In essence we become our own therapists.

To aid in this process I am including scripts throughout the book that you may use and make into recordings if you so choose. For those who don't have recording equipment cell phones may be utilized, then all you have to do is lie back with your head supported and listen to the soothing words.

If you don't enjoy the process – and hypnotherapy doesn't suit everyone – just count from five down to one, slowly, and tell yourself that by the time you reach the number one you will be wide awake. Then, open your eyes. For those who elect to make recordings, it is essential to only listen to them when you are relaxed and doing nothing else, listening while driving or doing other activities is dangerous as the hypnosis puts you into an altered state.

The scripts, also referred to as inductions, are generally in four parts. The first part relaxes your body and your mind and helps you enter the trance state in which you are more open to suggestions. The second part deepens the trance (this deepening is sometimes interwoven throughout the script) and the third part includes the messages you want to send to yourself: Healing messages of hope, strategies for dealing with treatments, reduction of stress, pain or anxiety and the wish for a healthy future. The fourth part is the counting out induction, which should be slowly read aloud, or otherwise you might get a headache. It is important to note that when a hypnotic script tells you to go into a deep sleep, it doesn't really mean fall asleep, it simply means relax your body. The only exception would be a script that is being used to help an insomniac get some sleep.

Reframing a situation is often helpful but you might wonder how cancer could be viewed as a gift? People with a diagnosis frequently ask, "Why me?"... I don't know why some people are afflicted and others not but in the case of my own life, I began to look for the positive things that cancer was giving me, rather than the negative and I think this is a helpful technique for many of us.

In my case the first positive was and is the ability to slow down. Imagine moving at an accelerated pace all your life. As a child my doctor referred to me as a racehorse because he saw me running everywhere. As I matured I had a sense of urgency, almost as if I had to cram as much as possible into my life. Time was of the essence and now in retrospect I wonder if perhaps some part of me knew what lay ahead. This feeling of being rushed and overwhelmed is something that is shared by many of us. Modern society is fast-moving and my clients often complain of having too much to do in a day and of feeling exhausted by the time they go to bed each night.

How wonderful then, post cancer (having elected to reduce my workload) it is to be able to get up when my body wakens naturally. There is no jarring alarm clock and I find it is a true luxury to open my eyes after sufficient sleep. Physical pains are minimized and I feel good, mentally and emotionally. Leisurely I watch the morning news with my husband, make a healthy breakfast, eat what I can, then set about to do the things I want to do with my day, not the things I previously had to do. Doing the things we like to do has a huge psychological benefit.

When I was in treatment I sat out in the garden and read for a while. We have been in our current home for twelve years and previous to my cancer (notice the possessive case) I never took time to sit in the garden. Now it was a pleasure to enjoy the flowers and watch the various birds that came to visit. Sometimes I just drifted off into space, and it was wonderful to have peace without the pressure of having to do anything in particular. Reading for pleasure was something I forfeited 30 years ago. Although I continuously read for my work there was never time to read just for enjoyment so the wonder of experiencing novels again was fantastic.

During chemotherapy going for a walk was a slow process as I couldn't move quickly. Prior to cancer, walks had consisted of my husband and I speedily marching along, taking large strides and thinking of the calories we were burning. Cancer allowed me to slow down and enjoy nature. To notice things that would never have caught my eye before, the different types of grasses, the way butterflies seemingly danced in the air with each other and the sun reflecting off the river like dappled, diamonds. My husband and I had time together to talk and enjoy mutual silence (wonderful when you feel very sick) and to do chores, which still need to be done in every household even when people are unwell. The difference was that we were no longer on a timetable. Saturday and Sunday were not the only days to complete endless chores. Being forced to slow down also gave me increased empathy and I was better able to relate to other people in similar situations.

Reflection was and is also possible, how many people get the time to enjoy memories of what has been and still have hope for what might lie ahead. Daydreaming is very underrated. To be able to get off the rollercoaster of life and pause is something not many people are afforded until they reach retirement. Up until this point I had studied hard, brought up four children and ultimately spent the majority of my life and energy working but when I became really sick it was my husband who truly supported me.

Family and friends were wonderful and all offered help but I was most comfortable in the presence of my husband. The realization that he was my rock and that I had been busy taking him for granted all these years was impactful. So one of the greatest gifts, love, had been with me all the time but I appreciated it with a freshness that was new.

My family life changed also because now I (as all mothers know we are generally loved but our efforts taken for granted) became the focus of attention. It was strange and touching. My youngest daughter whom for the last couple of years I managed to irritate by just being my own lovable self started being friendly again. She was patient and had time to talk to me and share her life and that alone brought great joy.

Another little pleasure, as mum I have always been the family photographer and as such tended not to be in as many photos as everyone else. But with the onset of cancer I was suddenly a star and everyone wanted to ensure that I was included in the pictures. So strangely another gift is one of appreciation. Ultimately cancer brought our family even closer. Initially we were shocked and upset but my family became very attentive and cancer made us more appreciative of the time we have together. Now we frequently have family gatherings and my youngest daughter has even spent time teaching me how to fish!

As I was bringing up our children when they were little, on occasions, I experienced a deep sense of loneliness. My husband, friends, family and career were unable to fill something in my soul, which was missing. At the time I believed it was the separation from my mother in Britain. Since developing cancer however, I noticed that loneliness has gone. My connection with God through prayer and meditation intensified and the deeper connection forged through the cancer, with the people in my life, has caused that loneliness to go.

The disease has also improved the quality of my work. Post cancer I chose to continue working in my practice part time, and I am now more compassionate as a counselor and hypnotherapist and no longer rushed. Ironically when things in life were full of hustle and bustle there was a sense of disconnection. However, now that I have had cancer everything has slowed down and I am again connected. Time is different-better and strangely I am happier.

Friendship wise I realized I had limited my social interactions with others to Xmas, Easter and holidays. Yet my friends were truly wonderful when they learned of my diagnosis. They emailed me, took me for coffee, kept my spirits up and distracted me from my fears. Suddenly I was aware of the quality of these relationships and how important they were in my life. When my health improved I intended to change my priorities and spend more time with family and friends and less time at work.

Perhaps the biggest change was the release of pressure due to the ability to slow down. My personality is such that if there's nothing to do I will create something.

Up till now, I had been a go-getter, a goal-setter, if I said I would do something, I did it. My jobs were demanding and I am a bit of a workaholic getting up at 5 am to prepare for clients and working till 10 pm some nights. I often saw private clients in the mornings at the office before going to school to work with teenagers during the day.

Afterwards, I rushed back to the office and continued seeing clients till late in the evening.

My career was demanding and time consuming leaving weekends only for my husband and family. Why did I do it? Two reasons, because I loved it and I wanted the money in order to travel.

Post cancer I am able to enjoy my work even more, and savor the experience. To sit with people, hear their stories and understand where their belief system comes from, why they see things the way they do, is fascinating.

I feel honored when they share their stories with me. To be able to help some of these people along the way is a privilege. I am amazed at the number of individuals in jobs as diverse as banking, engineering, and trucking who genuinely have a deep desire to help others.

Somehow, I used to believe that it was only the people in the helping professions (nurses, doctors, counselors, teachers) that had such motivation but that's not so. It seems to be a deeply human trait that the majority of people want to help others.

For me, being a counselor is who I am innately – I like people, I am naturally empathic and want to make a difference. In addition, I like to learn and find psychology, a variety of healing modalities and the realm of spiritualism fascinating.

My truest joy is the use of hypnotherapy to help people learn how to use their own minds for healing.

People say it must be a draining job but I find it energizing.

On weekends pre-cancer I enjoyed my down time with my husband and adult children. After completing some chores my husband and I would do something fun on a Saturday afternoon, perhaps a run to the States and a nice meal or a movie in the evening. Sundays were allotted to the kids, a weekly swim for exercise, a family dinner and other household chores.

All in all I thought I was compensating for my stressful weeks with my healing weekends. True, we relaxed (despite the endless chores) but I always felt very tired and at the back of my mind I wondered if I would be able to meet the following week's deadlines. Now those deadlines don't exist.

Another gift that cancer has given me is the satisfaction of slowly completing tasks that I wanted to do but never had time to do before. Of pursuing interests that previously remained on the back burner.

It's true that during school vacations I had a reduced workload, and I was able to rest more, although I still saw private clients.

The remaining time was taken up socializing with friends as well as family and enjoying my other great passion, travelling. I wanted to see as much of the world as possible.

Ironically, I believed I was doing all the right things to combat my fast paced, stress- filled life. I exercised, watched my weight, drank only occasionally – always just one glass of red wine – ate dark chocolate, took Calcium supplements, vitamins and oil, and relaxed as much as I could on weekends but it was not enough.

Cancer helped me to reprioritize my life, to create a healthy balance, to savor each day and to be grateful for what I have.

When we think of all the well-meaning advice we are given to "Be positive," perhaps there is a realistic way to do that. From a therapeutic stance it may be helpful to reflect on your life pre-cancer and post-cancer and see if you too can reframe what initially seems like a curse into a gift. Rather than dwell on what has been lost, which we all tend to do, why not look for what has been gained?

3: Treatment

And so my life changed dramatically. It went from working full time, half the week as a school counselor in an alternate program for teenagers, and half the week in private practice as a counselor and hypnotherapist, to no work at all. Treatment was essential and to be honest, initially quite daunting, so I decided to use the skills I had to support me through whatever harrowing experiences lay ahead.

First was the surgery, a lumpectomy or partial mastectomy and I made up a hypnosis tape, referred to as an induction (See Induction #5, page 79) to prepare my body so it would be relaxed during the procedure and heal rapidly afterwards.

I listened to the recording several times before the surgery and as a result felt much calmer on the day than I would otherwise have been and I knew that I wanted that tumor removed no matter what.

I am including several inductions in this book, which you may use to help yourself through treatments. They are all numbered and the pages given for easy reference however you can mix and match scripts depending on your preference.

If you wish to work on reducing a tumor using hypnosis before, during or after treatment, please use Induction #10, page 94.

As I lay in the prep area one of the surgery nurses, an older lady in her 50s approached me and said she had the same surgery ten years previously and had survived and been fine ever since. Her words really helped me and later when I saw her in the operating room I felt greatly comforted. What a wonderful thing she is doing by giving the gift of hope to frightened people. I cannot thank her enough.

Due to the skill of the surgeons and hypnotherapy my physical recovery was fairly rapid (See Induction #11, page 97) and it was soon time for the chemotherapy to begin. Now like everyone else I had watched many tear jerking movies with cancer victims undergoing chemotherapy, vomiting incessantly, (See Inductions #3, page 72 and #9, page 91) losing their hair and wasting away so this was not something I relished.

In fact, I was terrified and apart from praying, which has always been an integral part of my life I again prepared hypnotherapy tapes in advance. These were filled with suggestions that the drugs would target all the cancer cells, destroy them and ultimately leave my body cancer-free. In addition I worked on reducing my anxiety and seeing myself in the future, healthy and active. (See Induction #6 page 81)

I also spoke to people who had been through similar experiences. One of these women suggested I get a portacath implanted in my chest as she thought it was easier than having the chemotherapy administered through the arm. Furthermore, it meant I would be able to swim during the months in treatment – and since that is my favorite sport, I took her advice. Now chemotherapy is different for everyone but boy was I naïve to believe that I would even want to swim throughout treatment! Nevertheless the portacath was implanted and I was ready for the next stage.

My husband and two of my children came with me for the first chemotherapy session. The nurse explained that the effects were cumulative and the more treatments I had the stronger the impact on my body. On the plus side this meant that more and more cancer cells would be destroyed but unfortunately I would become weaker and more tired as the weeks progressed.

She said the symptoms felt a little like having the flu. It was with a great deal of trepidation that I entered the room, full of people silently hooked up to their chemotherapy drips, and received my first dose of the medication.

To me the whole situation was incredulous. I couldn't believe that I was a cancer patient. It didn't seem possible. It was also a little embarrassing for me to see my children watching their mother suddenly helpless when the image I had always tried to portray was one of strength. Now here I was in this awful situation.

When the drug entered my body I tensed waiting for an immediate negative reaction but of course the effect was gradual. Only at the end of the session did I notice a difference. I felt dizzy and lightheaded as if I'd had too much wine but without any joyful intoxication.

Chemotherapy continued for 12 weeks, it should have gone on longer but my body could not tolerate the second drug I was supposed to take. I was therefore given a choice, try a different drug or stop chemotherapy. I chose the latter.

During the chemotherapy treatments I also had to administer a drug by injection (See Induction #4, page 75) for a few days between treatments. Being faint of heart I elected for my husband to pierce my skin as the thought of doing so myself was too much. Now Roy doesn't have the best eyesight so the first time he gave me the vaccination in my stomach, supposedly subcutaneously, I thanked him. I said it barely hurt and that I would pump the syringe liquid in myself as I wasn't sure how it would feel. Surprisingly the syringe plunger seemed to resist the downward pressure and eventually liquid began to dribble out onto the surface of my skin! I was puzzled until I realized that although Roy thought he had inserted the needle, it had not gone through the skin's surface, which is why it didn't hurt! From then on I injected myself and now have great compassion for diabetics who have to go through this procedure daily.

The final part of treatment was radiation, which I received daily for 6 weeks. (See Induction #7, page 85) Again, hypnotherapy was utilized and this time I envisioned the radiation destroying the cancer cells – while an invisible coating protected the healthy cells. The process was time-consuming but the hospital staff was wonderful. During the initial visit a cast was made so that my body would always lie in the same position for each treatment.

After a while, my cast became uncomfortable and my arm went numb and cramped but when I told the technician he explained that it was probably because I had been in it too long and the actual radiation sessions would be shorter. Despite his reassurance, I was anxious that my arm would cramp and I would have to move suddenly especially in the initial treatments. Thanks to hypnotherapy however I was able to reduce my anxiety and allow my body to remain motionless during all of the sessions.

Each treatment brought with it different challenges: After surgery my body was sore to the touch (See Induction #8, page 88) and the arm was weaker where the lymph nodes had been removed.

The hospital gave me a list of gentle exercises to be used throughout the following weeks and wanting as much mobility as I could get I diligently carried them out.

My breast also felt sore and after the surgery I couldn't even look at it let alone touch it. The idea of its deformity repulsed me and to actually view it made the reality of the cancer more intense. Somehow by not looking I could pretend that things were not really so bad. Like the ostrich putting its head in the sand.

Eventually, about six months after surgery, I addressed the problem and desensitized myself by looking at the breast with a small shaving mirror, a little at a time. In the end I was able to look at the area in detail and accept the new me. By then the tissue had filled out somewhat and the deformity did not look so awful.

Next, slowly and with some dread I very gently touched the area and continued to do this daily until I was able to overcome my own aversion and accept the changes. Those baby steps were milestones for me.

Throughout I continued to listen to my healing inductions (See Inductions #12, page 100 and #13, page 104) and when I was not in the comfort of my own home, I often practiced self-hypnosis (See Induction #20, page 124) to promote healing.

In therapy a Gestalt technique to help release suppressed emotions, which may create physical and mental pain, is to talk to parts of your body. After a pause you then imagine becoming that part of your body and correspondingly respond. For instance, if you feel angry and notice that feeling seems to be stored in your stomach you then dialogue with your stomach. It appeared to help many of my clients so I began using the process myself and held conversations with my breast. I thanked it for all it had done, for feeding my children when they were young. The right breast for some reason was the favorite with all 4 of my children – and I told it how sorry I was for the present situation.

I imagined my breast replied by telling me not to blame myself. I apologized by saying that my overworking probably contributed to the onslaught of this disease and that from now on we would work together towards better health. I also explained that the treatments were a necessary part of fighting the disease and that we were a team, body, mind and soul. All intertwined in the struggle for survival. Simultaneously I was using a pain induction (See Induction #8, page 88) to help my body feel better and after a while, using both techniques, the pain subsided.

Some people view cancer as the body attacking itself but I chose to see the body as my friend, we were/are a team with the same ultimate goal, health and survival. Although I blamed myself for the onset of my disease (by overworking and neglecting my health) there are many people who do everything correctly, they eat well, sleep well and exercise well but still become sick.

I realize that there are so many different types of cancer and we are still trying to understand a variety of possible causes. It's extremely important therefore that individuals do not blame themselves for creating the disease when in all probability they are guiltless. This book is not meant to set a standard of how to sojourn through the disease. It is simply a true account of my experiences and of the things that helped me. You the reader should take what is useful and discard the rest.

As a youth I believed that I would reach a ripe old age as a fit and healthy senior. When I saw older people who were not fit I erroneously assumed they had not taken care of themselves properly.

As I matured my perception changed and I became aware that a healthy body is not simply the result of living a healthy lifestyle. Genetic predisposition, disease, accidents and a multitude of unknown causes all play a part.

During the chemotherapy part of my treatment my energy level was so depleted, the only way to help myself was via a combination of meditation, prayer and hypnotherapy (See Induction #12, page 100). Treatments took place in the summer months so I was able to go outdoors with my husband and take a short walk most days. Leaning heavily on his arm and taking mincing steps with many breaks along the way, we headed towards a bench by the river where we could sit and enjoy nature.

At times it was difficult for me to open my eyelids as the energy required seemed too much so on these snail paced walks onlookers were probably convinced that I was dying.

The effort was great but well rewarded as the peace and beauty of our natural surroundings was very healing. The fight to maintain some level of daily energy led me to have great empathy for the sick, the dying and the elderly.

Admittedly the doctor told me I'd lose my hair temporarily and although he assured me that it would grow back and I tried to tell myself that it was not a big deal, the reality was quite different. For me at least it turned out to be a very big deal.

By the second chemotherapy treatment my hair started to fall out en masse, I brushed it and a whole lot of hair remained on the brush, I gently tugged and the hair came away in my fingers. Heartbreaking and devastating!

When you've spent 62 years styling, brushing, and rinsing these tresses it definitely makes an impact as they begin to shed.

Suddenly I was faced with this awful realization that the worried face in the mirror was me. There was no soft hair to cushion the blow, just the bare, hard fact that this sick, bald-headed, old face belonged to me. In that moment I became painfully aware of my own mortality. I couldn't even bring myself to look at my bald head until after I underwent the third chemotherapy treatment.

For years I had subconsciously associated a cancer victim's baldness with the horror of the German concentration camps and the word cancer itself instilled great fear. To look at cancer patients sporting baldheads was repugnant and something I had avoided at all costs. Now that image was my reality!

Somehow I had to come to terms with the pain and distress so I decided to start by buying a wig. It was very expensive but fortunately extended health covered the cost. However it didn't look natural to me so I bought a scarf and attached a small patch of hair, resembling bangs, to the front so that it looked as if I had tresses. Initially my head felt itchy but vanity is a great motivator and after a few days the discomfort passed.

It's strange how we always want what we don't have. The hair on peoples' heads became my focal point and in restaurants and other public places I studied everybody's hair with great fascination and envied their haute coiffure.

At home, meanwhile, I knew I had to come to terms with my new baldness so I took a shaving mirror and studied my hairless head from all angles. It was very strange.

At first my repulsion was strong but every night before bed I would take that mirror and look at myself from every angle until eventually ugly and vulnerable gave way to sadness and acceptance. Slowly I managed to desensitize myself.

After a couple of months of chemotherapy I no longer had enough energy to talk to people I met in public situations like shop clerks or bank tellers.

Normally I have a cheerful, friendly disposition and chat to most people I meet, just pleasantries. My world therefore was a warm reciprocate place, I smiled at someone and he or she generally returned the compliment. When you show an interest in people they open up and become communicative. During chemotherapy however, I stopped making conversation unless absolutely necessary as it was far too draining.

To my surprise the majority of people were not comfortable initiating small talk so my public world became colder and more distant.

Like many people I am a placator (people pleaser) and it was important to me to be liked and make people feel comfortable, usually by initiating conversations. I noticed nevertheless that others did not do this and many silences ensued.

Suddenly I was very aware of how much energy I had expended each day trying to make others feel comfortable and that alone time for reflection had practically been nonexistent.

At this point I also found the smell of my own body offensive. Sensitivity to odors has always been a trait of mine and chemotherapy seemed to heighten it.

Perfumes and aftershave, used (excessively at times) by the young adults in my house practically knocked me out with their intensity.

My own scents became too much, what had once been pleasant now turned my stomach. I was afraid to use the underarm antiperspirant, which had been my friend for 40 years (because I heard that it might lead to breast cancer).

So, I instead tried a natural crystal product with a lavender smell. Of course it didn't work as well as my antiperspirant. Not only did I feel hot and sticky but the lavender smell made me nauseous and I began to associate the body odors and perfume with being sick. My solution was to avoid perfumes and wear natural unscented deodorants.

Later however, my oncologist told me there was no evidence to suggest that antiperspirants increase the risk of breast cancer, so I have reverted back to using antiperspirants.

The final part of treatment, the radiation, was lengthy but due to a glitch in the system I had a longer time between treatments and felt a little better.

Continuing to use meditation, prayer and hypnotherapy was helpful and I also started trying to swim again. The hot tub was my incentive, as the warm jets of the water seemed to ease my stiff joints. The latter was a side effect of the chemotherapy and although I swam very slowly, I still rewarded myself both before and after the experience with a relaxing time in the hot tub.

4: Anxiety and Depression

When I started treatment I did not have a fear of needles (See Induction #4, page 75). Eventually however after much prodding on my left arm (the right one could not be used since the sentinel nodes had been removed during surgery) and despite the portacath I began to dread blood work and IVs. In fact fear (See Induction #3, page 72) and anxiety became my bedmates and I was also afraid of the chemotherapy. Sure it could destroy the cancer but what else might it destroy? I began to dread the hospital environment and when it came time for radiation I was worried about the damage that might be done to healthy tissue. At night I would waken up in a sweat (no doubt a reaction to the chemo) and once I cooled down, I could not get back to sleep again. Terrifying questions ran through my mind. When would I die? How would I die? What would it be like to die? And what happens after death? Needless to say I spent many sleepless nights until I began to use hypnotherapy to ease the anxiety and fear (See Induction #2, page 69). Convincing my subconscious that all would be well was just the panacea I needed.

Reading or going on the Internet is informative but during my illness I had to be careful because having too much information was dangerous. First of all there are a lot of contradictory ideas about how to deal with cancer and there are a lot of horror stories. So I would read about the importance of one diet then read about a completely different approach. Being suggestible and having a vivid imagination is good for hypnosis but dire warnings about side effects from treatments made me very nervous and afraid that I would have a negative reaction of the worst kind. (See Induction #1, page 65)

When my radiation finished I was told that it was in my best interest to take a hormone pill for the next five years. This created more anxiety because I went on the computer and read the reviews of people who had taken the drug and of course some responses were negative. As a result I limited my reading, particularly about procedures I had to undergo, until the night before the actual event. In that way I also limited my anxiety. I believe that it is important to know your facts because we have to advocate for ourselves and our loved ones therefore a certain amount of knowledge is necessary. For example I knew that it was important to drink plenty of water when undergoing chemotherapy and fortunately I did. It wasn't until near the end of treatment that a nurse told me I could have developed cystitis If I hadn't followed protocol, so educating yourself is both motivating and helpful. Of course some people are just too anxious and would rather bury their heads in the sand and pretend the whole thing isn't happening and that is their choice. We all have to cope in the best way we can.

Even though I was in the middle of this crisis the rest of my family could not totally smooth the waters around me since they themselves had to deal with the shock of my disease and their own life stresses. During chemotherapy my oldest daughter broke off her engagement with her fiancée and came back home to live, in a very distraught state. At the same time my second daughter and her husband had been living in the States but the military lifestyle put a strain on their marriage and sadly they decided to separate. As a result Heidi returned home to Canada with her five-year-old son. My youngest two were already living at home so the house was filled to capacity, which at times was both a blessing and a curse. On the bright side I had many distractions to keep me from focusing on myself but on the other hand my children's suffering was painful and upsetting. As they say, "Into every life a little rain must fall." At the time it seemed more like a deluge! It was interesting because I actually felt physically sick to my stomach when the stress became too much so using the following inductions (See Inductions #14, page 108 and #15 page 111) was particularly helpful in these instances.

Normally for my type of cancer it's about 3 weeks between chemotherapy and the start of the next phase of treatment, radiation. Considerably weakened both physically and mentally by the preceding weeks I did not feel ready to cope with this final onslaught. Fortunately, at least from my perspective, there was a delay as the doctor's referral did not go through in a timely manner and so I had a few extra weeks to get stronger.

As the months passed my two oldest again moved out of the house and once more there was a semblance of calm at home.

Ultimately I was given the all clear, the treatments were over, the mammogram didn't detect any lingering cancer cells and the oncologist said I was cancer-free. Relief was immediate and we all celebrated by going out for dinner.

In my case, although I felt better I still did not feel great or like my old self, and that's when the doubts began to set in. Was I really cancer free? Were there any malignant cells hiding in my body, as yet too small to be detected by medical technology? Was it going to come back?

These thoughts flooded through me and I feared and began to believe that I only had a maximum of five years left and perhaps even less than that. As a result I spoke to others as if that belief were a fact and privately became very afraid.

Slowly, imperceptibly, a change came over me, and in the mornings I awakened feeling flat and joyless and realized this could lead to depression (See Induction #16, page 113) if I didn't do something about it.

Depression (See Induction #17, page 116) is quite common after being diagnosed with cancer and undergoing treatments so I knew that it was a real possibility. Sometimes we hold on so tight, fighting the disease and when it's all over we relax and boom it hits us. At other times we become depressed during treatments.

Naturally I turned to my hypnotherapy and made up a variety of recordings, emphasizing insight and inner resources, which could be utilized to aid in recovery. (See Inductions #18, page 119 and #19, page 122).

Listening to these tapes repeatedly over several weeks helped calm my racing thoughts and lightened my moods. Ultimately they prevented me from falling into a deep depression, which could have robbed me of precious time. It takes an encounter with cancer to make you appreciate the moments of your life.

Although I do not belong to any particular religion, spiritual churches have always intrigued me. I was aware that on certain days of the month mediums frequent such churches and give readings to some of the members in the audience. To aid in my healing I decided to go to one of these sessions with my husband and see if I was lucky enough to get a reading.

Secretly I was hoping that my mother would come through and tell me that everything was going to be alright just as she had done when I was a child and needed comforting.

The message from Robin had helped tremendously but now I needed another boost. Begrudgingly my husband came with me (he is not as open to the idea of the dead relaying messages from the other side) and we sat in the congregation. There were two mediums on stage and they took turns channeling messages but as the evening wore on and the end was almost in sight neither of them had directed their attention towards us.

Fortunately, just before the end, one of the mediums pointed to me and said he had a lady beside him that he thought was my mother. I was thrilled (no one in this church knew about my cancer) and he went on to say that she was showing me her bruised arm as proof of her identity. Immediately I knew that it was her. During her life my mother had a heart condition and consequently needed to give blood samples at the hospital every month. Unfortunately she was put on an anticoagulant and the medication caused her to bruise easily so by showing me her arm she was confirming her identity.

The medium continued to give me messages from my mother, which were accurate and then seconds before the end he said. "She wants you to know that you still have a long time left!" That was the message I needed and wanted to hear.

Throughout treatment I had exercised whenever possible and eaten as well as I could but now the determination to eat healthily and exercise more strengthened. I joined a stretch and strength class, went for a daily walk and swam twice a week. Fresh vegetable and fruit became an integral part of my diet and I cut back on red meats and sweet treats. As a result my mood brightened and I began to enjoy life again.

5: John of God

I first heard about John of God, 15 years ago when I was looking through some DVDs at work. He is supposedly one of the most powerful channeling mediums and healers alive today. Intrigued I asked a few people about this man and shortly thereafter viewed the DVD. It was fascinating, in front of my eyes I saw him perform strange surgeries with no anesthetic and the subjects appeared to feel no pain. On some occasions a surgical clamp, which looks like a pair of long forceps, was pushed down the noses of individuals and turned repeatedly and these people did not even squirm; others were surgically cut with knives yet showed no sign of discomfort. Next were interviews with people who swore that they had been cured of a variety of ailments and the film was very convincing. But of course the camera can lie and so although I was left wondering about the validity of the whole situation life continued and I eventually forgot about John of God.

A year later after my diagnosis and treatment for cancer I still, on occasion lay awake at night wondering: "Will it come back? Am I really cancer free?" The events that happened next were serendipitous. As mentioned previously every now and then I attended a local spiritual church. On one of those visits I was lucky enough to hear a speech given by a woman who had gone to see John of God because she had been suffering from breast cancer. Years later she remained cancer free and credited this to his treatments. I began to wonder... then, strangely, while at work I met a new (to me) counselor called Peggy, who was also an energy healer. We were both waiting for our next clients and had some time to chat. "How do you actually do energy work?" I asked. Peggy laughed at my curiosity and said, "Let me show you. Let me take away the pain from your neck and back." I was surprised that she knew I was experiencing such pain. In fact from time to time, when stressed I did experience tension in those areas but I never mentioned it to anyone. So, having it pointed out was a little unnerving. Nevertheless with 10 free minutes to spare before my next client arrived I agreed to let Peggy energize me. Her movements were odd as she wove around my body seemingly pulling out things invisible to the naked eye but and here's the wonderful part, my pain (all but one spot the size of a teaspoon) completely disappeared and I felt relieved. "Wow, thank you that really made a difference." I said. She smiled and replied, "Ever since going to see John of God my healing powers have increased." "Oh you've been there have you?" I asked incredulously, "I'd love to hear about your experience…" my voice trailed off as my client arrived. "Yes of course whenever we get time," said Peggy and she hurried away however it would be several months before we again met up.

In the interim one of my friends, Laurie was having physical pain so I referred her to Peggy and not only did Laurie get better but the two women became good friends. Peggy's enthusiasm and conviction about John of God led Laurie ultimately to make the trip to Brazil. She was on a spiritual quest and came back enthused and a total believer.

Apparently the first time Laurie, who is extremely sensitive to energy, waited to view John as he entered the great hall she suddenly felt intense vibrations travelling through her body. These almost caused her to pass out and she slid down the wall towards the floor. Luckily, two women helped her but as a result Laurie missed the entire event! I listened eagerly to the accounts she and Peggy relayed and made my decision: We (my husband and I) were going to Brazil!

In December of 2015 we flew to Brasilia, stayed overnight and were picked up the next morning by a driver who took us to Abadiania, a small town about one and a half hours from the capital. Our group leader Heather Cumming had arranged everything for us. When we arrived at our destination we were welcomed into our hotel and introduced to the other guests all of whom had come to see John of God. They were having lunch and we joined them and were invited by Heather to go to the waterfall that afternoon for a spiritual cleansing. I had read about the waterfall before making our trip and I knew the water would be icy cold particularly since my friends had also warned me. My husband on the other hand, had no idea and was surprised by the temperature! Later we both agreed that after our long, hot, trip and that initial cold shock, the water was very refreshing.

John, João de Deus, visits his healing center, the Casa de Dom Inacio, often simply referred to as the Casa on Wednesday, Thursday and Friday. This meant we had time on Tuesday to explore the region around our hotel and we found lots of small stores selling local crystals and jewelry. It was very hot and a little like walking back in time, so different from the high rises and modern buildings in North America. I wondered if the streets of Bethlehem, around Jesus' time, might have borne some resemblance to Abadiania.

Back at the hotel we listened to stories of miraculous healings performed by John and told to us by the other hotel guests. One elderly gentleman had been in a wheelchair, five years previously and his wife persuaded him to visit John even though he was a non believer. Reluctantly he agreed thinking, "Well I have nothing to lose." and lo and behold John worked on this man and then told him to get out of his wheelchair and walk. Amazingly he was able to do so and has not been in the wheelchair ever since but he visits John from time to time because it makes him feel good!

During our stay another individual in his eighties, a retired doctor, was feeling very ill and his wife was afraid she was going to lose him. Heather took this gentleman to see John privately and during the healing the doctor said he felt as if his whole stomach was moving up and down quite violently. It was as if he had washboards in there but when the movement stopped he felt much better and continued to feel better for the duration of his stay. In fact the next day was the Christmas party and the old gentleman was out with the rest of the group enjoying the festivities.

On Wednesday we went down to the *Casa* and there were literally hundreds of people waiting to see John. We all wore white clothing since it is easier for the Spirits of Light who work through John of God to see the body's hologram and blueprint if white is worn. From what I understand, John channels one of thirty three entities, beings that have lived on earth before and come back to help people who are sick and suffering from a variety of ailments. While living on the earth they were apparently doctors and healers and there are thousands working invisibly at the Casa. However there is always one, who, using John's body, directs the proceedings of the day. John has been working at the Casa for over thirty years and he is free of charge so the Casa makes its money by selling herbs, and blessed items and artifacts.

The quiet seriousness in the main hall, made a great impression upon me. There were prayers being said in Portuguese and sometimes in English. Soft music played and although the Casa welcomes all religions it combines Spiritism, with Catholicism and the atmosphere was very soothing. Without pomp or ceremony I saw John walk up to a woman who was standing against the wall. He moved his hand in front of her stomach and her chest and I assumed he was anesthetizing her energetically. John then took the long forceps and moved them down into her nose and twisted them round and round. She screwed up her eyes but did not scream or shout out in pain. Eventually he removed the forceps and there was some bloody tissue attached to the instrument. Later on I asked Heather what he had removed and she said it is all energy work. Next John turned to a gentleman in a wheelchair and began to scrape his eye with a knife. I anticipated what would come next (because of the DVD viewed previously) so I closed my eyes and did not watch the entire procedure. The man in the wheelchair however was apparently ecstatic after his treatment as witnessed by some of our group who sat beside him in the main hall. After this John went to sit down and we, the masses patiently waited for our turn to file past him.

Prior to visiting the Casa we were allowed to list 3 things that we would like healed, in order of priority. Our leader said it could be an emotional, physical or spiritual issue and she promptly recorded these. Personally I thought this was rather amusing like giving God a shopping list and expecting him to fill it. Nevertheless since remaining cancer free was my main reason for making this pilgrimage I too made my requests. The idea was that when our turn came we were to file past John and our leader would go up to him with this information. As Joao does not speak English Heather would relay the information in Portuguese and he would tell her what kind of treatment we needed.

Some people were waiting in line-ups, standing for a long time while others like myself were afforded the luxury of a seat. It was interesting looking around the main hall, there were a few babies dressed in white, but most of the people that day were adults young and old, some obviously very sick. What struck me was the fact that everything seemed very genuine and I heard that John had been doing this for a long time and was now in his seventies.

I was calmly sitting watching the hundreds of people pass by the healer and waiting patiently for my turn to see him when I remembered my friend's reaction to Joao's entry into the hall. She felt intense vibrations moving through her body and almost fainted, and I thought to myself how melodramatic Laurie had been because I was not aware of any supernatural happenings.

No sooner had that thought entered my mind when all at once large spherical lights so bright, so white, so painfully blinding, flew towards me at great speed as if entering my body. My head and neck felt intense pressure pushing downwards and my skin became hot and clammy. It was shocking and I knew I was about to pass out so I touched our leader who was standing beside me and told her. She acted very quickly and in what seemed like an instant I was in a wheelchair being pushed past hundreds of people waiting to see John of God. " Keep your eyes open!" Heather (our leader) kept telling me and I did but the brightness of the lights was painful. Suddenly there I was face to face with John of God, Heather knelt by his side and spoke to him in Portuguese, presumably explaining why I was there and he conversed with her. I looked into his eyes, which were filled with compassion and mentally said, "Thank you." and then it was over.

The whole experience seemed momentary and in an instant I was outside in the shade, still in the wheelchair, slowly recovering from my ordeal. It took a little time for me to realize that what I had probably experienced were the entities of light and that they had already started working on me. It was a humbling experience, a miracle, one that I will never forget and for which I am eternally grateful.

The next day we began our treatment set out by Joao and my husband and I were told to each have a spiritual massage that was to last for 90 minutes. Now this was a bit worrisome as my breast, underarm and arm were still tender from the surgery and I was afraid massage would be uncomfortable however I was wrong. The whole process was extremely relaxing and pleasurable, not at all like the deep tissue massages I had endured in the past.

After this we were told to book a couple of crystal bed sessions which involved lying on a bed, underneath healing crystal lights and listening to relaxing music. The crystal beds help rejuvenate, align and balance our energy fields and the crystals act as a portal for the healing entities. For me the session brought up sadness as I relived the trauma of my diagnosis, the tests and the treatments so it was cathartic. After the sadness I felt extreme peace and moved into a deeply meditative state.

My husband felt nothing but peace and said he fell asleep for a short time. One of the other people in our hotel told me that each time he lay in the beds he felt anger so I think that whatever is needed in that moment is what people will experience.

We were assigned a specific time and day, for our psychic surgery and in the meantime were encouraged to sit in Current, that is, one of the meditation rooms alongside many other people. Sitting in the current is both an act of giving spiritual energy and receiving it. The term "Current" refers to the spiritual energy generated by people who meditate in the room and is used by the healing entities. Apparently it can raise one's vibration and allow everyone to act as channels of energy. I do meditate but not for long periods of time so after one and a half hours I left the hall but some people sat for much longer.

On the third day we had our intervention or psychic surgery and joined hundreds of people in a large hall to receive our healing. We simply closed our eyes, said a prayer and put our hand over our heart, remaining that way for 15-20 minutes.

After the intervention we were prescribed medication in the form of capsules (containing Passiflora, an herb derived from passion flower that had been blessed by the entities) and then ushered out to a waiting car and taken back to the hotel. Even though we had no incisions made on our bodies we were told that it was essential to treat our psychic surgery the way we would treat a physical surgery by letting our body rest and slowly repair itself.

At the hotel we were instructed to go to bed for 24 hours and to take a vow of silence so that recovery could be enhanced. Apparently most people sleep for the duration wakening only at mealtime if desired. My husband did just that but I was awake for about 7 of these hours and found it a little difficult since we were not allowed to read, or write during this time.

A week after the intervention we were asked to wear white at night, leave a glass of water by our bedside and say a prayer. It is believed that the entities come and take out any internal stitches that one may have received during the intervention. Taking the pills three times a day until the prescription runs out is also a requirement and participants are told not to eat spicy food, drink alcohol, or have sex or any other form of intervention for 40 days.

Exercise is also discouraged for the first 8 days and then we are encouraged to have a gradual return to our individual routines.

A week later both my husband and I were back home, we felt better and there were physical changes. I experienced less body pains and my husband's tired legs were re-energized.

Looking back I believe that something miraculous happened to me. Of course, I hope I am cancer free, but even if I am not, the journey itself was both amazing and healing and the rest is up to God. My energy although not what it was pre-cancer is good enough to let me do everything I want to do, albeit at a slower pace.

Now I am not advocating that anyone who gets a cancer diagnosis should run out and book a ticket to Brazil. That is just not feasible. This is simply the story of my journey and the things that have helped me on the way.

The fact is that many people go to John of God and are cured while others are not. Although I believe that death is simply a transition from this world to the next and that passing over is not necessarily something we should fear I still have reservations and want to spend as much time on earth as possible.

Knowing that our minds are extremely powerful and have a definite impact on our physical wellbeing it is important to work on keeping calm and remaining optimistic.

As cancer patients we are all on a journey (admittedly not one we would have volunteered for) with limited options. We either give up or cope with it in the best possible way, with hope, faith, humor, courage and all the tools we can muster!

6: Going Forward

How to make the best of the time left? That's truly the conundrum, dilemma and challenge that faces all of us after a diagnosis of cancer.

Once all the treatments are over it is possible to just enjoy the moments day-by-day hoping all will be well. Of course it might be, but for me, my bout with the disease was an awakening, which made me aware of my own mortality and how precious life is. This in turn caused me to prioritize and evaluate through reflection and meditation, what I'd like to do with the rest of my life.

I felt a deep sense of gratitude. I'd been given a reprieve and consequently needed to give back in some way. After much consideration I decided to run a small hypnotherapy group for people who had cancer, those who were undergoing treatment and those who were cancer survivors.

The first group ran for 6 weeks and consisted of inductions geared towards dealing with cancer treatments and general healing. I fully intended to repeat the same material every two months with a new and different group however my second group wanted to continue meeting so that's what we have been doing for the last 2 years.

Over these years participants have come and gone but four have endured and they've taught me as much as I've taught them. The group has evolved into one of sharing and supporting each other as well as a place where members are hypnotized and record the inductions on their cell phones.

During the course of our sessions it became apparent that we had all dealt with our cancer diagnoses in different ways and I asked each member if they would be willing to share what had helped them in their fight to survive. Fortunately all agreed and perhaps their experiences will help you the reader in your journey. Before engaging in any treatment including hypnotherapy, however, make sure you first talk to your medical practitioner and become well informed.

The first member of the group, Deborah, is a married woman with two young boys who was diagnosed in her fifties, with ER+ (estrogen-receptor positive) breast cancer. This is the most common type of breast cancer and one, which responds well to treatment with hormonal therapies. The oncologist and surgeon told Deborah that she had to have a full mastectomy and would require chemotherapy and radiation.

Their recommendations however did not sit well with Deborah's own belief system. Deborah preferred less invasive treatment and wanted to have a lumpectomy, followed by a course of natural healing. When her initial oncologist made the above suggestions Deborah felt as if her body was screaming out, "No! No! No!" so she did some research and found an oncologist and surgeon whose beliefs matched her own.

"We get so frightened as cancer patients and believe that we must immediately do what the doctor tells us to do," Deborah said. "But we don't have to. We have to feel right about the course of action inside ourselves and find doctors that are a good fit for us."

Deborah's cancer was stage 2 and had not spread so she felt that it was not a panic situation and her advice to others who find themselves in similar circumstances is to relax and research. Deborah had to wait two months for her surgery and was told by the initial surgeon that if she refused conventional treatment her cancer could grow and she might die.

Nevertheless, Deborah ignored the surgeon's warnings and followed a natural course of action by changing her diet. Over the next two months her tumor size did not increase. Happily, Deborah's surgery was a success, and although the oncologist wanted to do radiation therapy just to make sure no malignant cells were left, Deborah declined and instead fully immersed herself in natural treatments.

Believing that cancer could not grow in an alkaline environment she changed her diet completely and consulted an herbalist/nutritionist to help her make the transition. Deborah's diet was mostly vegan, and she avoided anything that would increase the estrogen in her system.

Her naturopath encouraged Deborah to try an alternative therapy called oxygen therapy, which is based on the premise that oxygen kills cancer cells. She taught Deborah to increase her intake of oxygen by doing specific exercises, deep breathing, drinking alkaline water and by participating in ozone therapy. The latter floods the body with oxygen and may be administered through an intravenous line or by removing the blood, oxygenating it, and returning it to the body. If you use this type of therapy it's important to find a qualified practitioner, as the procedure could be harmful if improperly administered.

In order to drink alkaline water Deborah and her husband researched which kind of filter would be suitable. They decided on a Life Ionizer, which claims to raise the pH of water (making it alkaline) by using electrolysis to separate the incoming water into acidic and alkaline components and remove toxins from the water. She said the water's so pure it's as if it's straight off the mountainside. She drinks

15-20 cups a day because her body craves it, and it tastes so good. More information on alkaline diets and alkaline water may be found on the BC Cancer Agency's website.

Deborah visited Inspire Health, a nonprofit organization in Vancouver, which supports people during and after cancer treatment and is approved by the BC Ministry of Health. She found their rehabilitation services were great and that they offered exercise therapy, stress management, nutrition and counselling all free of charge. Deborah was given a lot of information, met various professionals, attended exercise and cooking classes and was offered nutritional plans, which enhanced what her own nutritionist was suggesting. In addition they had weekly meditations that could be done over the phone and that was very useful since Deborah lived a distance away from the premises and at that point in her recovery she was still in a fragile state.

For a year and a half Deborah was very strict about her diet, so the change was drastic and she ate only organic food and no genetically modified grains. It was a challenge, but she enjoyed making, "a home for healthy cells." She meditated on a daily basis and received massage at West Coast College of Massage Therapy in New Westminster. Treatment was provided by students, training to become massage therapists. This made it more affordable.

Support was very important to Deborah. Her husband, and most of her friends and family provided this. But she was surprised that some people she thought would help did not and others she didn't expect would help, did.

For people without family and friends in the area, Deborah suggests joining one of the many support groups in the lower mainland. Deborah's husband was very good at researching cancer and its various treatments.

Even so, Deborah admitted that her experience was initially overwhelming and the treatments, herbs and foods were expensive. Despite this she is now cancer-free and her advice to all cancer patients is: "Don't panic just educate yourself."

The second member of the group, Ivy, is in her sixties and was first diagnosed with breast cancer in 2004. In 2008 she was given the all-clear, but sadly the cancer returned six years later, as stage 4 and had metastasized into her bones. When Ivy learned she was cancer-free she didn't do anything different to maintain her health as she was already living a healthy lifestyle and, was working and busy.

From the time of her second diagnosis, Ivy has been participating in a volunteer program at the Cancer Clinic where she takes trial drugs and is consistently monitored. She takes these drugs to help further research and to benefit future cancer patients. She is giving back in her own way and is currently on a trial drug, which has been approved in the States. Ivy considers herself in remission because in the last four years her cancer hasn't spread. "I think I am in a holding pattern." she says. Ivy has tumors on her spine but deems herself lucky because she feels no pain. Before her diagnosis she was not overly stressed and does not believe that stress played any part in causing her illness.

When Ivy was re-diagnosed she didn't look for any outside resources as she was busy caring for her husband, who had been diagnosed with Alzheimer's and this preoccupied her time. When he passed, the next year was a blur so a friend took Ivy on a trip to Europe, a very pleasant distraction.

For the last 10 years Ivy has belonged to a book club and to keep her mind active she attends a night class in winter, and takes online university courses, which are free, unless you want the credits.

Throughout, the most important things for Ivy have been her faith in God and the support of her family. Ivy's advice is: Keep busy and distract yourself. In the group we find she exudes a quiet calmness, and an acceptance of what is while still remaining bright and optimistic about the future.

The third member of the group, Linda, was diagnosed in her fifties with cancer of the right breast and she had a mastectomy followed by chemotherapy and radiation. Unfortunately the chemotherapy was too strong and Linda ended up in palliative care in hospital and almost died. On recovering she chose to have the other breast removed because she thought the prosthetic would be uncomfortable and she opted to have breast reconstruction. A year after diagnosis Linda was given the all clear and remained cancer free for the next six years.

In 2016 the cancer returned and metastasized to her bones so Linda was put on a trial drug, which was unsuccessful. The doctors then wanted to put her back on the same drug that previously made her sick but instead Linda sought a second opinion outside of the BC Cancer Agency.

She found a naturopathic doctor who had a Hyperthermia machine from Germany. This machine directed heat (high energy waves) to the tumors on her bones near the body surface, killing the cancer cells. After one month of 12 treatments all the spots were gone. This naturopath also referred Linda to a medical oncologist who prescribed different medication and Linda says these two treatments saved her life. Now Linda's cancer levels are consistently low and the doctors say it is 'like' being in remission without actually being 'in' remission. Linda has blood tests every two months and she lives a healthy lifestyle. For anyone interested in using Hyperthermia be sure to learn about the possible side effects of this treatment.

Linda told me about Callanish, a community-driven group based in Vancouver that helps people who are living with or dying from cancer. The organization offers retreats, counseling, meditation groups, family support and craft programs. Linda also takes yoga at a seniors centre.

She says there are many meditation groups in the city to choose from and activities for fun, like laughter yoga are offered through meet up groups. Her advice to others is don't be afraid to get a second opinion regarding treatment and be proactive. Look at what's available and learn as much as you can in order to make informed decisions.

The fourth member of the group, Alex, in his fifties, was diagnosed with stage 4 Non-Hodgkin lymphoma (NHL) in 2016. He underwent chemotherapy and received a stem cell transplant. This involved stem cells being introduced into his blood intravenously, similar to a blood transfusion. The procedure enables stem cells to go to the bone marrow and produce healthy new blood cells. Alex is still receiving chemotherapy and will do so for the next two years.

Although the cause of most lymphomas is not known he says that he was very stressed the year prior to his diagnosis and thinks this might have played a part in causing the disease. His wife has been the one to research and glean as much information as possible on NHL. Meanwhile Alex prefers to know just enough of the facts as he deems necessary. In this way he has been able to reduce his own anxiety and remain optimistic. When he has the energy Alex loves to play tennis and spend time with his family and he is currently cancer-free.

Alex appreciates each day and his advice to others is "Don't sweat the small stuff, take it easy and enjoy life."

Perhaps the most encouraging account comes from Judy, a woman who was diagnosed in her forties with breast cancer and is still alive and in good health 28 years later. Admittedly the cancer did resurface in her other breast two years ago but she has had it removed and is again cancer free. My daughter worked with Judy and asked if she would be willing to share her story with others, fortunately she agreed and talked to me by phone.

Apparently Judy initially had a lumpectomy and some lymph nodes removed back in 1990 and at that time patients were kept in hospital for a week in order to recover.

Unfortunately, the day before she was to be released the surgeon told her she needed to have her whole breast removed. As you can imagine that was quite a shock for Judy but she had no choice other than have the mastectomy and stay in hospital for another week.

After surgery, she went on a course of chemotherapy administered by shots and while she was on chemotherapy, which can lower your blood cell count and cause serious complications, Judy took Royal Jelly and Ginseng Pills. She believes these kept her platelet count at a healthy level. Although this helped Judy it is essential to first consult with your medical professional and become informed as to possible complications before taking any natural health products during treatment.

When chemotherapy was finished Judy took Tamoxifen, a hormone therapy drug, taken in pill form, to block the actions of estrogen. Luckily she was able to tolerate the drug well and stay on it for five years. The doctors would not allow her to have an implant for those five years. In fact it was closer to ten years before she had one, so Judy used a prosthesis during that time. When she was first diagnosed

Judy had been a social smoker but she quit immediately upon learning of the cancer and has never smoked since.

Judy was and is a very energetic person. While receiving treatment, and still bald from chemotherapy, her husbands' two children came over from Chile to stay with the family for several months. Judy was able to take care of them in addition to her own three children and after treatment she worked hard holding down three jobs. "I was a real tough mom," she says, "because I had been divorced and wanted my daughters to be strong, independent women who would survive even if something were to happen me." As it was everything worked out fine in the end.

Over the years Judy has spoken by phone to women who have received a breast cancer diagnosis and has helped alleviate some of their anxieties. She is not religious in the sense of going to church regularly but she believes in a power greater than self and this faith helped in her recovery. When asked how she would advise others Judy said: "Keep busy and be optimistic, a positive mindset is important."

Knowing how other people cope with and survive cancer is very helpful for everyone who has received a cancer diagnosis. Throughout my journey I had been keeping a diary and the process of journaling was very therapeutic. In time I realized that sharing my experience might be beneficial to others. If something good could come out of my ordeals then my suffering would not have been in vain and so the idea of writing this book was born.

Now coping with cancer is one thing but what to do after treatment is over and how to live a fulfilling life is in itself a conundrum, a challenge and it will be different for every individual.

For me, enjoying my family was paramount, helping the children establish themselves and sharing in their joys and sorrows was a given but what else should I do? I thought of travelling around the world, it's something I had always wanted to do. Such a trip however would take us away from the family and my practice for too long and it would wipe my husband and I out financially. All our life savings would be gone and there would be nothing left to buffer us against the harsh realities of life. Ironically I might even live until I am 80, anxious and in poverty.

On the other hand if my death was imminent, what a regret to think that such a trip was never made. A compromise had to be reached, a balance created, but creating such a balance was easier said than done. There was also the question of work, for us money is and will always be an issue, after all, the mortgage has to be paid. Should I work a 40-hour week or should I retire and work part time? Questions, questions, questions. Not being clairvoyant and knowing that time is precious I had to make a plan and hope for the best.

Admittedly, living in the moment and focusing on the day is important and many people choose to live that way. They enjoy and accept life and don't set themselves up for disappointment if plans fall through. But for me some sort of direction was needed since I am a planner.

Knowing I could die sooner rather than later is in a strange way, a kind of gift. When you actually think about it not many people are given that information but cancer patients are only too well aware of their possible expiration date.

Realizing that time is of the essence can mobilize each of us into action to ensure that whatever time is left is wisely used. I asked myself, "What matters most? How should I utilize this precious commodity of time?"

In therapy we tell people to savor the moment, become fully involved in whatever they are doing, be it eating an apple or lecturing from a podium and we call this mindfulness. I wanted to do that and more, I wanted to sit down, survey my life and decide what things gave me the most pleasure and incorporate these into the remaining days, weeks, months and hopefully years.

In addition, I noted the things I hadn't done that were important and still possible for me to do and made a mental list of which people I wanted to see more often.

Having a large pension to take care of me in my old age was now less important, after all there are no guarantees in life so money took on a slightly different flavor.

It's true we all need enough money to survive but spending the majority of time accumulating wealth no longer held any appeal.

Every day in the news we hear of people dying sometimes a few sometimes many. What made me any different? Nothing, we are all human beings vulnerable to the laws of nature and the acts of man. The only difference was I had been told that my time may be short. I had been warned.

So what matters most? I meditated on this for quite a while and the answers that came to me may be similar or quite different from yours, or other readers.

For me, it was clear that people, family and friends were top of the list, my bond with loved ones and the interactions I had on a daily basis with others preceded all else. Realizing this I then examined the experiences in life that had given me the most pleasure and those were being out in nature, skiing, and surfing, horseback riding and playing with my border collie. The first three had an element of speed about them and the latter two involved animals. Finally as previously mentioned, I had always enjoyed travelling and there were many places not yet seen so visiting different countries held great appeal.

As a result my bucket list had to incorporate all of the above to some extent. Since I already lived with my family and enjoyed my friends and interactions with people at work, increasing these aspects of my life was all that was needed. Being out in nature is also easy when you live in a beautiful area like Vancouver, which is surrounded by water and mountains.

Since my body was no longer fit enough to participate in the sports I liked due to the cancer and also to osteoporosis, a speedboat or sea doo might give me the thrill I wanted. Playing with a dog could easily be accommodated and travel was a possibility. Like many women I got a thrill out of clothes shopping. Although it seemed foolish to accumulate clothes that might only be worn for a short time the joy came from the hunt as well as wearing something I loved. Process as well as fashion! While our bodies are well we have a choice ruminate and brood or make the most of the situation and live. I chose the latter.

Perception is everything, viewing each day as an opportunity to be enjoyed held more appeal than the alternative and this was my gift, appreciation of the value of life and of time. I had appreciation for what I already had and what I could still do.

In the Storyteller by Jodi Picoult the grandmother has had a mastectomy and her granddaughter sees her naked in the shower for the first time. Instead of hiding her body the old lady is open about the situation and says: "But see how much of me is left?" What a wonderful attitude.

When I had recovered sufficiently, I wasted no time and decided to quickly visit all the places in Europe that I hadn't seen and still wanted to. As a result, my husband and I went on a marathon tour, which included parts of France, Italy, Greece and Britain. Marathon because neither of us was in the best of health and the trip involved hours and hours of sightseeing, most of it on foot. Needless to say we were totally exhausted at the end of the month but it was wonderful and had I died immediately thereafter it would have been fine since my wanderlust was satisfied.

Nevertheless as all seasoned travelers know, although it's great to get away, and lovely to return home, within a few months that urge to explore reappears and the desire to globe trot resurfaces.

I pondered the situation for a while and alighted upon the idea that two or three trips a year could be a good solution to creating a balanced life. One trip to enjoy the sun and escape dreary winter weather, another to visit family and friends in Britain and one to explore countries yet unseen.

Now this all sounds very glamorous and extravagant but truthfully because of age and health we cannot know how many trips we will actually be lucky enough to take. So I decided to strike while the iron is hot and hope for the best.

After much thought, I opted to retire from my counseling position with the school board. Instead I would just keep my private practice, working reduced hours, a couple of days a week. That way I could regulate the number of hours I worked according to my level of energy. Cancer changes us forever on so many different levels and how we change internally is quite fascinating and uniquely individual.

Ten years prior to my diagnosis we had moved into a new house and were able to furnish it the way we wanted. Up until that point most of our furniture had been secondhand and well used by our four children so this was a fresh start.

I took great pains to ensure that everything matched color wise and the outcome was a well furnished, comfortable, very conventional home. I had a green and gold bathroom with matching towels, bathmats, and all the accessories. Everything flowed. Nothing shocked the eye.

Post cancer, I decided to add a dash of color and brighten up the place. My pale lemon floral wreath was replaced with a bright splash of lime and my soft green candles that surrounded the bathtub gave way to luminous lime!

For the first time in my life I had the confidence to express myself and show my true taste. To make decorative changes all through the house, not simply follow what I deemed to be socially acceptable.

My taste in clothes also changed: Before getting sick I enjoyed wearing bright colors but during my illness I wanted to wear darker fabrics and soft gentle colors. Now, after recovery, I enjoy both bright and subtle colors.

Being faced with the possibility of imminent death spurred me on to do the things I had always wanted to do but never got around to. I attended a developmental circle in a spiritual church to heighten intuition, attended healing touch classes and learned how to do stage hypnosis for fun.

In fact, the cancer experience is almost contradictory: In one way it makes me want to glean everything I can from life and in another way, I want to give back. Both drives are equally strong. Each day I try to be mindful at least part of the time, making an effort to enjoy the fact that I'm still here.

7: Inductions for Fear and Anxiety:

Receiving a cancer diagnosis may initially produce extreme anxiety and fear. I remember the moments after being told that there was a lump in my breast first experiencing disbelief, followed immediately thereafter with a terrible sense of dread. My heart was pounding in my chest and, I felt light headed and found it hard to breathe, all symptoms of anxiety. If you the reader feel highly anxious and afraid then the following inductions may be helpful.

Read the induction first to get a feel for it, and then record the words, speaking slowly and clearly into the microphone. Inductions should never be listened to while driving or operating machinery, as you will go into an altered state. Instead find a quiet and comfortable place where you can relax. Loosen any tight clothing, remove glasses or contact lenses and ensure that your head and neck are supported. The reason for the latter is that when you relax deeply your head may fall to one side and pull on your neck. It is also important not to lie flat as this makes it easier to fall asleep and unless that is your objective an upright position, whether sitting or lying down is preferable.

1 Anxiety Induction and Imagery.

Find a comfortable place to sit down and make sure your head and neck are supported then relax. Close your eyes and begin to take slow, deep breaths. Imagine that someone is touching the middle of your forehead with his/her finger and still with your eyes closed look up to that spot on your forehead. Now count slowly from 1-5 and say the word "Sleep." between each number then notice how very comfortable your body is beginning to feel.

Cancer Conundrum / Louise Evans

When you reach the number 5 relax your eyes and imagine yourself standing in a beautiful old English garden. It's a warm summer's day not too hot, just right for you and you enjoy the warmth of the sun on your skin, caressing your body. The fragrance of your favorite flowers, subtle and pleasantly soothing fills you with delight and you look around the garden at the myriad of blooms, every type of flower imaginable. Mostly domestic varieties but there are a few wild flowers scattered here and there, dancing in the gentle breeze. There are trees and shrubs and grasses, freshly fragrant on this summer's day and every shade of green imaginable. You touch a flower's petal and marvel at the velvety soft texture of the plant, so delicate and so beautiful. The birds are singing in the garden, some of them happily splashing around in a small fountain and you notice with interest that there is no one else in this garden. This is your special place, a place of peace and serenity. To the right is a small naturally occurring spa bubbling up from the ground below and some part of you realizes that these are healing waters and you watch with fascination the fine mist which forms above the surface of the water. There are large white fluffy towels beside the spa and the noise of the bubbling water and the slight smell of the naturally occurring minerals are soothing to you.

In a moment I'm going to allow you two minutes of clock time, all the time in hypnosis time that you need to enjoy your garden and then I'll resume talking again. I won't tell you what to do, you may enjoy walking around and exploring your garden, or sitting or lying down and looking up at the cloudless sky above or you may watch, paddle or bathe in the healing waters of the spa. Whatever you do it will be most enjoyable and you will drift deeper and deeper into comfort and trance.

The silence that follows is the deepening and then the following suggestions are given.

Imagine that you are sitting in a beautiful old theatre with comfortable, plush velvet seats and a large red velvet curtain overhanging the stage. All around you people are talking quietly, then the orchestra begins to play, and as the music fills the room the curtain rises and an expectant hush falls over the audience. The curtain moves slowly upwards revealing actors and actresses on stage, all brightly dressed. You lean forward in your seat and listen intently as the characters come to life and create a storyline, which amazingly seems to mirror your own worries and concerns. It's incredible that the issues they are dealing with are the same issues you are dealing with. What a strange feeling to see your problems externalized, almost as if they were performing this play just for you. You watch closely as the plot unfolds.

Pause for two minutes to review before continuing.

Act one is over, the curtain falls and the audience applauds then the hall fills with noise as people get up out of their seats for the intermission but you sit motionless savoring the moments. Soon break time is over, the curtain rises and once more an expectant hush falls over the audience. Everyone is wondering how the characters will resolve their issues. What strategies might they use? Initially they try one course of action, then another and another, mesmerizing the audience with their ingenuity and variety of possibilities and always demonstrating the likely outcome of such actions. Solutions are being played out in front of you, some you had already considered and others that are new to you and all you have to do is watch.

Allow a two-minute pause in your recording in order to view the scenes.

Finally the play ends with a standing ovation and you are delighted because now you have more ideas on how to solve your problems. In the days that follow and in your dream cycles your subconscious mind will continue to help you with creative ideas and allow you to feel calm and relaxed.

In future if you experience anxious thoughts in your head, you will hear yourself shout, "Stop!" loud and clear, "Stop!" And this is a sign to distract yourself and redirect your thoughts to something more pleasant, more peaceful, a time when you felt calm, relaxed and very, very good.

It might be a memory from childhood or it may be more recent. If nothing comes to mind you can use a favorite daydream or a fantasy. An idea will pop into your mind easily and you can take your time and enjoy the sights, the sounds, the scents, the flavor and the feel of that situation. And as you do so a deep sense of peace and a feeling of wellbeing permeate every cell of your body and you feel safe and relaxed, safe and relaxed as you savor the moments.

Use the counting out induction below to return to full conscious awareness. As always, this should be read aloud slowly, otherwise you might get a headache.

Now enjoy your special place for a few moments longer then I am going to count from five down to one and when I reach the number one you will come back to full conscious awareness feeling very, very good.

Five*, you have done some good work today and you are learning how to use the power of your subconscious mind to help and heal yourself.* ***Four****, each and every time you choose to do this kind of therapy, whether with me or another hypnotherapist or listening to your recording you will go deeper and faster than the time before.* ***Three****, you will gain great healing benefits and enjoy the process immensely.* ***Two****, slowly, gently, normal sensation returning to your body and you may wiggle your fingers and your* *toes and* **One,** *returning to full conscious awareness, aware again of the sounds in the room and eyes open wide, wide, wide awake feeling absolutely marvelous. And if you like you can give yourself a positive mental suggestion as you reorient back to the room.*

The first part in italic type takes you into trance and the final paragraph in italic type is the counting out induction, which may be used at the end of each induction to bring you back to conscious awareness.

2 Anxiety Induction and Relaxation.

This should be read very slowly and is not suitable for anyone with a fear of water.

Take a nice deep breath, close your eyes and begin to relax and just imagine a beautiful waterfall cascading down into a tropical lagoon below. It is nighttime and the sky is a velvety black, the stars sparkling like tiny diamonds embedded in its smooth surface and the air is pleasantly warm, as is the water. You sit by the edge, feet dangling in the lagoon and watch the water, silver in the moonlight, flowing endlessly down, down, and down, deeper and deeper and deeper. The movements are mesmerizing and you relax even deeper, relax even deeper. The occasional sound of a distant animal is surprisingly soothing and you have a sudden urge to enter the water and swim towards the cascading liquid. It feels warm and comfortable and you watch the silver ripples emanating from your hands as you move silently through the liquid. There is something so healing about the experience that you swim for what seems like a long time and then venture towards the edge of the cascading falls and let the waters gently shower over you. Amazingly it is just the right temperature and as the water caresses your body it creates a deep sense of peace and relaxation. It flows over your head relaxing all of the little muscles in your scalp and face, over your shoulders and arms, like a soothing balm. Down over your chest and stomach, warm and relaxing and all you have to do is think about relaxing those muscles and they will relax. As the flow continues, down, down, down, over your legs and feet, it creates an even greater sense of relaxation and eventually you swim lazily to the edge of the lagoon, dry yourself off with a nice white fluffy towel and lie on a nearby hammock looking up at the stars above. The hammock rocks to and fro, to and fro, to and fro and you find yourself gazing lazily at one particular star, the brightest and the biggest and as you do you go deeper and deeper relaxed. Enjoying the peace and quiet, nothing to think about, nothing to do but just lie there and relax as if you are floating on a sea of dreams, enjoying calming thoughts, peaceful thoughts and you can remain that way for some time as you drift deeper and deeper into total relaxation.

Allow 2 minutes of silence then resume talking.

Now that you are so deeply relaxed your subconscious mind is open and receptive to suggestions, which are all for your benefit and you realize that there are many ways to let fear and anxiety dissipate. Imagine for a moment that you can feel the exact location of the anxiety in your body. Notice what it feels like… Does it vibrate through your body, feel scratchy or rough, is it subtle or harsh? Take your time and become aware of the feeling.

Next, notice if it has a color. Is the color light or dark and what shape is it, round, cylindrical, square or rectangular? Notice also how big it is.

Perhaps your anxiety has a sound, perhaps it resonates like the beat of a drum or squeals like a piccolo, maybe it shrieks like an untuned violin. Whichever way you experience anxiety I want you to imagine letting it go in whatever way feels right for you. If your anxiety resembles the noise of a practicing orchestra, whose musicians are unskilled and whose instruments need tuning then you may simply let go by changing the music. Allow the musicians to harmonize and create a beautiful symphony that moves through you like a wave of relaxation and calm. If it feels harsh and physically uncomfortable you might imagine letting it go as a blanket of warm tranquility wraps around you and the vibrations and roughness melt into the fabric. If it has a color perhaps you'll see the color rising up and out of your body. Moving further and further away, higher and higher until it disperses into the atmosphere and is completely gone... And all the cells of your body are soothed and comforted as if you are being rocked in the arms of a safe and nurturing mother.

Slowly... gently... you leave the hammock, walk to the edge of the lagoon and stare at your reflection in the water. A beam of energy from above fills the areas that were anxious with a glowing, pulsating light, and this grows stronger and more vibrant with every passing moment. Peace, tranquility and courage fill you and you know that a power greater than self is helping. Deep gratitude flows out of you like a fountain spilling its waters endlessly while the light continues to replenish your entire body. You feel safe, so safe and there is a deep sense of peace that permeates every cell, every fiber of your being and grows stronger and stronger as you relax deeper and deeper.

Note. *If you are listening to this recording at night and want to go to sleep, the induction could end here or you could use the counting out induction below if you wish to rouse yourself.*

Now enjoy your special place for a few moments longer then I am going to count from 5 down to 1 and when I

reach the number 1 you will come back to full conscious awareness feeling very, very good. **Five**, you have done some good work today and you are learning how to use the power of your subconscious mind to help and heal yourself. **Four,** each and every time you choose to do this kind of therapy, whether with me or another hypnotherapist or listening to your recording you will go deeper and faster than the time before. **Three,** you will gain great healing benefits and enjoy the process immensely. **Two,** slowly, gently, normal sensation returning to your body and you may wiggle your fingers and your toes and **One,** returning to full conscious awareness, aware again of the sounds in the room and eyes open wide, wide,wide awake feeling absolutely marvelous. If you like you can give yourself a positive mental suggestion as you reorient back to the room.

3 Combating Fear

Before using this induction make sure you are sitting upright with your head and neck supported.

Start by putting a coin between your thumb and index finger and hold your arm out in front of you, with your wrist facing downwards.

Now focus all of your attention on your thumbnail and don't let your gaze move. As you do so you begin to notice the coin is feeling heavy. Notice also the different sensation in the tips of the fingers, they might feel hot or cool, heavy or light, tingly or tremulous. As you continue to focus on the nail the eyelids become heavier and heavier and your eyes may begin to water. Just a little at first until eventually they close and then you can imagine a wave of relaxation moving through your body. Slowly the coin begins to feel even heavier and heavier and eventually it slips gently through your fingers and falls to the ground below. When the coin hits the floor that is a signal to your subconscious mind to enter trance and to allow a second wave of relaxation to pass through your body. Now your arm feels heavy and tired and you can slowly move that arm down towards your lap and as it touches your lap you can go twice as deep as you were before.

Next take 5 slow, deep breaths and with each exhalation you find yourself drifting deeper and deeper into comfort and trance until after the fifth breath you are very deeply relaxed. 1 inhale slowly, filling your lungs with air, hold this... and as you exhale release all the stress and tension and slip deeper and deeper into relaxation 2 inhale deeply, hold the air... and as you release feel yourself sinking down and down, more and more into a state of quiet tranquility 3 take a deep breath in, hold it... and as you breathe out blow away all the worries and cares of the day 4 inhale deeply, hold the air...and as you exhale go deeper and deeper relaxed and 5 inhale, hold the air ... and as you let it escape, feel yourself move all the way down, all the way down into a very peaceful state of relaxation.

We all experience fear at various times in our lives, sometimes a little and sometimes a lot. When fear becomes unmanageable it can paralyze us and impede healing but there is a way to reduce fear and cope more effectively. Start by externalizing your fear by giving it a size, shape and color and then put that image several feet in front of you.

 Now look at your fear, study it while still maintaining a safe distance between it and yourself. Whenever you feel afraid imagine creating a beautiful aura of protection around your body. Maybe it's a glowing white light, a soft pastel shade or a vibrant color, whatever you wish and this acts like a warm soothing blanket surrounding and protecting you. Next begin to remember a time you felt truly loved. Remember that person in your life who loved you and joyfully bring that memory to life. Relive it, every detail, enjoy it, see it and feel it and as you do so the aura around you grows stronger and the fear diminishes (pause for 1 minute). Remember cuddling a new born baby, a child or a beloved pet. Feel the physical contact, the warmth, the sensation of comfort and well being – the pleasure of connection. Allow all of your senses to indulge in the moment (pause for 1 minute) and as you do so the aura around you grows stronger and the fear diminishes.

Now move in time to one of your happiest childhood memories. For some people it's seeing a particular flower for the first time or getting a puppy or winning an award, it really doesn't matter what it is as long as it makes you happy. Spend time enjoying that memory (pause for 1 minute) and as you do so the aura around you grows stronger and the fear diminishes

Next remember a spiritual experience that filled you with peace and joy. Perhaps it was religious in origin, perhaps it was marveling at the beauty of nature, the wonder of the stars and planets in the universe, perhaps connecting with whatever you believe the divine to be. Again it really doesn't matter what it is so long as it feels good to you. Spend time enjoying that memory (pause for 1 minute) and as you do so the aura around you grows stronger and the fear diminishes.

Think of all the things that you are grateful for now and in the past, the things you've seen, heard, smelled, tasted, touched, the people you've loved and those that have loved you (pause for I minute). And as you do so the aura around you grows stronger and the fear disappears.

Now enjoy your special place for a few moments longer then I am going to count from 5 down to 1 and when I

reach the number 1 you will come back to full conscious awareness feeling very, very good. **Five***, you have done some good work today and you are learning how to use the power of your subconscious mind to help and heal yourself.* **Four***, each and every time you choose to do this kind of therapy, whether with me or another hypnotherapist or listening to your recording you will go deeper and faster than the time before.* **Three***, you will gain great healing benefits and enjoy the process immensely.* **Two***, slowly, gently, normal sensation returning to your body and you may wiggle your fingers and your toes and* **One***, returning to full conscious awareness, aware again of the sounds in the room and eyes open wide, wide, wide awake feeling absolutely marvelous. If you like you can give yourself a positive mental suggestion as you reorient back to the room.*

4 Needle Phobia Induction and Progressive Muscle Relaxation

During treatments it is often necessary to give blood samples or have medication administered by IV and for some people the anticipation of this is unsettling and arouses fear. Using the induction below you may become more relaxed with the process.

Sit down in a comfortable chair, with your head and neck supported and take a nice deep breath, inhaling through your nose for the count of 4.... holding the air for 4 seconds... and exhaling slowly through your nose... Imagine that you are breathing in peace and tranquility and breathing out stress and tension. Do this again, slowly inhaling ... holding the breath... and slowly exhaling through the nose.... Notice how comfortable your body is beginning to feel. And again inhale... hold... and exhale... With each exhalation you become more and more relaxed.

Finally one more deep breath inwards.... hold the air for 4 seconds... and as you release it feel your body move even deeper into comfort and relaxation.

Now imagine your favorite color starting as a wave of relaxation at the top of your head and slowly moving down through your body to the tips of your toes.

As it moves down it touches and relaxes every part of your body and the more relaxed you become the better you feel. All of the muscles in the scalp and neck begin to relax as that beautiful color touches them and as the color moves down over the face all of those muscles begin to relax and let go. The forehead smooths out and relaxes and even the tiny muscles around the eyes, the nose and the mouth release and let go. And as this happens you move deeper and deeper into comfort and trance.

Now that beautiful color moves along the shoulders and into each of your arms. See the bicep muscles tight, taut and tense and the moment that color touches them they let go and relax. Then the color moves down through the elbows and around the elbows and into the muscles of the forearms and these muscles let go and relax and you go deeper and deeper into comfort and trance. And the color moves into your hands and out through your fingertips so now you have a wave of relaxation moving from the top of your head, across your shoulders, down both arms and out through your fingertips.

Take another nice deep breath as the color moves into your chest and your stomach relaxing all the muscles there. At the same time imagine a wave of relaxation moving down your back, down, down down, to the lower part of your back. These muscles let go and with every breath you exhale you slip deeper and deeper into comfort and trance. The beautiful color continues to move downwards through your hips and yours thighs and notice what it feels like for the thigh muscles to let go and relax. The color moves down each leg around the knees and through the knees and into the calf muscle. Again imagine these tight, taut and tense and the moment that color touches them they release and let go. Now the beautiful color moves into the feet and out through the toes and it is as if the feet have been tightly bound and the moment the color touches them they are able to spread out and relax. And now your whole body is deeply relaxed as this wave of relaxation washes over and through you from the top of your head to the tips of your toes.

And from your place of peaceful relaxation take a nice deep breath and begin to use your imagination. Imagine placing your hand in a bucket of ice-cold water. At first your hand tingles with the change in temperature and as you leave it in the bucket, it gets colder and colder, colder and colder, number *(pronounced nummer)* and number, until all sensation disappears and it becomes totally numb. **Allow enough time for this to happen.** Now remove that hand from the bucket and place it on the area that the needle is to be inserted into. By transferring all of the numbness from the hand (so that the hand again feels normal) to the needle site, you are anesthetizing the area and there will be no discomfort during treatment. After treatment normal sensation will gently return to the area.

And while the needle or IV is inserted imagine being involved in an activity that you enjoy... perhaps it is swimming or cycling... or doing photography...or just going for a leisurely walk along a quiet path in nature. Notice how pleasurable it is pursuing something you enjoy, something over which you feel a sense of mastery, notice every detail. Your body is familiar with the activity and your mind is relaxed so you can just savor the moments **(pause for 1 minute).**

Feel that sense of well being in your body, all through your body. The next time you feel any fear around needles notice where in your body that fear is and simply remember your enjoyable activity, remember every detail and transfer the feeling of comfort to the place in your body where you previously felt fear.

Now enjoy your special place for a few moments longer then I am going to count from 5 down to 1 and when I reach the number 1 you will come back to full conscious awareness feeling very, very good. **Five**, *you have done some good work today and you are learning how to use the power of your subconscious mind to help and heal yourself.* **Four,** *each and every time you choose to do this kind of therapy, whether with me or another hypnotherapist or listening to your recording you will go deeper and faster than the time before.* **Three,** *you will gain great healing benefits and enjoy the process immensely.* **Two,** *slowly, gently, normal sensation returning to your body and you may wiggle your fingers and your toes and* **One,** *returning to full conscious awareness, aware again of the sounds in the room and eyes open wide, wide, wide awake feeling absolutely marvelous. If you like you can give yourself a positive mental suggestion as you reorient back to the room.*

8: Inductions During Treatment:

As cancer patients it is easy to feel vulnerable and helpless. If the disease is advanced treatment generally follows rapidly and we are encouraged to act quickly and follow the conventional path of surgery, chemotherapy and radiation. Not necessarily in that order. For those who choose this path, the inductions below will be empowering. You will move through treatment with a sense of wellbeing, knowing that you are utilizing the power of the subconscious mind to overcome the challenges ahead and aid in your recovery. Once again remember to read these inductions slowly whilst making your recordings.

5. Surgery:

Imagine yourself in an enchanted garden surrounded by your favorite flowers and your favorite colors. Perhaps there are hundreds, perhaps thousands, all in the bud stage. You walk over to the plants and examine one bud, its petals tightly closed around each other, the delicate stalk and the adjoining leaves. "If only they were all in bloom, how beautiful the garden would be." You whisper this under your breath and no sooner do you make that wish than all the buds in front of your eyes miraculously begin to open together, slowly unfolding their petals, like time-lapse photography. The garden swells with color and fragrance fills the air. A kaleidoscope of color surrounds you and you lie down on a grassy bank immersed and intoxicated by nature's beauty as a wave of relaxation moves through your body. You remain motionless for some time spellbound with the peace and tranquility of the garden and as you do so you begin to drift into trance.

Allow 2 minutes of silence before resuming the dialogue.

*Dreamily your eyes alight upon a tiny seed case attached to a little white parachute from a dandelion puffball and you watch as it floats down softly from above. You count the number of seconds it takes to reach the earth and as you focus on the white feathery tuft and count, you slip deeper and deeper into hypnotic sleep. By the time the chute lands on the ground you will be in a deep, deep, sleep. **1,** it wafts gently in the air, down, down, down, a delicate miracle of nature. **2,** it's so light, so quiet – soundless in its journey. **3,** deeper, deeper, deeper relaxed. **4,** it's floating and drifting on currents of air. **5,** now it reaches its destination and lands gently on the earth as you fall into a deep, deep sleep.*

And as you sleep you dream it is the day of your surgery and you feel calm and relaxed, calm and relaxed because the doctors are going to remove the unhealthy tissue from your body. You feel good because once the unhealthy tissue is removed you can begin to recover and you know that the surgeons are skilled and capable, capable and skilled. You trust their expertise and your body and mind are relaxed. The surgery goes well, everything proceeds as planned and soon very soon you are in the recovery room and the doctors are assuring you that the procedure went well. Relieved you go home and start to recuperate and in the weeks that follow the doctors are amazed at the speed at which your body heals. You are on the road to recovery and you can relax and let go, just relax and let go.

And now let your mind drift to a happy time, a time when you felt peaceful and relaxed. Perhaps it was at the beach on a hot summer's day after exerting yourself by frolicking in the ocean. Tired but content you lie down in a hammock and gently move from side to side, from side-to-side enjoying tranquility and peace. Or, maybe it's lying in a lover's arms while he or she softly runs his/her fingers through your hair or gently massages you.

The caresses take you into a wonderfully relaxed state, like a baby safely swaddled in his/her mother's arms, snug and secure, cozy and warm, listening to the lullaby she sings, as they rock back and forth, back and forth, back and forth. Whatever your memory notice every detail of that time, the colors, the fragrances, the sounds, feel the peace, spreading through your body, nothing to think about, nothing to do just let yourself be, immersed in tranquility and peace.

Now enjoy your special place for a few moments longer then I am going to count from 5 down to 1 and when I reach the number 1 you will come back to full conscious awareness feeling very, very good. **Five***, you have done some good work today and you are learning how to use the power of your subconscious mind to help and heal yourself.* **Four,** *each and every time you choose to do this kind of therapy, whether with me or another hypnotherapist or listening to your recording you will go deeper and faster than the time before.* **Three,** *you will gain great healing benefits and enjoy the process immensely.* **Two,** *slowly, gently, normal sensation returning to your body and you may wiggle your fingers and your toes and* **One,** *returning to full conscious awareness, aware again of the sounds in the room and eyes open wide, wide, wide awake feeling absolutely marvelous. If you like, give yourself a positive mental suggestion as you reorient back to the room.*

Remember, the first part in italic type takes you into a trance and the final paragraph in italic type is the counting out induction, which may be used at the end of each induction to bring you back to conscious awareness.

6 Chemotherapy.

This induction is easier to carry out if you are sitting in an upright position with your eyes closed. To start, stretch your arms out in front of you with your fingertips lightly touching the material of your clothing and your elbows out to the side of your body. Now take a nice deep breath in and relax and as you do so notice the texture of the material beneath your fingertips and the sensation in your fingertips. Imagine that there is a string bracelet tied around each of your wrists and radiating from those bracelets are silken strands all being pulled upwards by a charm of hummingbirds.

Feel the string around your wrists and see the vibrantly colored hummingbirds. Take another deep breath in and as you do notice a feeling of lightness developing in one or both of your hands. Watch those hands and notice that the right hand may feel lighter than the left or the left lighter than the right or they may feel equally light... it really doesn't matter, all that matters is that you feel comfortable and allow this lightness to continue.

Keep watching your hands at all times and soon you may notice that one or both of those hands begin to move upwards slowly, gently at first as if they are being pulled up by the birds, up and up, lighter and lighter, higher and higher. The hands may move up a little at times and then back down and then back up again and that upward movement may be tremulous and staccato like or continuous and smooth. And as those light hands lift higher and higher take in another deep breath and relax even more enjoying this feeling of lightness and upward motion. And the lighter they feel, the more they rise and the more they rise the lighter they feel. As this happens you feel more and more relaxed.

One hand may move quicker than the other or perhaps both move at the same speed It really doesn't matter all that matters is that you feel comfortable. And when your unconscious mind is ready for you to enter into a deep trance one or both of those hands may touch your face.

*When that happens, those hands may gently and slowly begin to move down towards your lap, taking you deeper and deeper into comfort and trance. And from your place of quiet relaxation you find yourself on an imaginary journey safely floating up through the blue skies to the clouds above and as I count from one to ten you continue to float even higher and drift even more into comfort and trance. **1**, you're becoming lighter and lighter. **2**, ... **3**, floating upwards **4**, ... **5**, more and more relaxed. **6**, ... **7**, floating and drifting, drifting and floating **8**, ... **9**, ... and **10**, so deeply relaxed and now you can safely float on your cloud for a while and look at the landscape below. Imagine the sounds, the smells, and the feel of the various places you float by as you continue to drift deeper and deeper into trance, drifting to the level that's ideal for your work today.*

The night before your chemotherapy treatment you will have a sound and restful sleep, a sound and restful sleep. On the day of treatment you will waken feeling calm and relaxed, and allow any negative emotions, doubts, stresses, anxieties and anger to release from your body, just let them go, let them float, far, far away. See yourself seated comfortably in the hospital ready to get your first treatment and feel a deep sense of peace and relaxation wash gently through and over you. Remind yourself that these drugs are your friends, your army if you like and it is their job to target and wipe out the unhealthy cells, to destroy them and restore you to good health.

Give the cancer cells a shape and a form and then visualize your army of drugs, soldiers and warriors perhaps, entering your body, finding the cancer cells, attacking them, battling them and ultimately destroying them. Imagine your white blood cells devouring the dead cancer cells and any remaining waste being excreted through your feces and urine. The medication has annihilated, the cancer cells. And the sound of my voice and each inhalation takes you deeper and deeper into comfort and trance.

While you sit there and the medication is being administered you might like to imagine leaving your body and travelling to a time in the past when you felt happy. Physically comfortable and healthy, a pleasant time where you can enjoy the scents, colors, textures and sounds of that time. Perhaps a day at the beach, the warmth of the sun on your body, the sound of the waves washing against the shore, a gentle breeze moving through your hair, the salty fresh smell of marine air and the silkiness of the sand against your skin. The feeling of comfort intensifies and to your amazement you find that real time passes very quickly and soon you are able to leave the clinic and go home.

At home as you rest on the sofa you project yourself into the distant future and see yourself at age 80. Your features are still recognizable although your hair is a lot greyer and you've probably gained or lost some weight as you aged.

Now, ask that 80-year-old all the questions that are on your mind and pause long enough after each question to listen to the answers. How did he/she survive the chemotherapy, what were his/her secrets, what did he/she eat, how did he/she deal with the nausea, the loss of appetite, the temporary change in energy and other side effects? What lessons were learned?

Some of the answers may not come immediately but ideas and responses will continue to come to you in your waking and sleeping hours. You see yourself as a survivor, able to overcome all challenges. Your desire to live activates your own healing resources, which continue to grow stronger and stronger as you grow healthier and healthier.

Now enjoy your special place for a few moments longer then I am going to count from 5 down to 1 and when I

reach the number 1 you will come back to full conscious awareness feeling very, very good. **Five**, *you have done some good work today and you are learning how to use the power of your subconscious mind to help and heal yourself.* **Four,** *each and every time you choose to do this kind of therapy, whether with me or another hypnotherapist or listening to your recording you will go deeper and faster than the time before.* **Three,** *you will gain great healing benefits and enjoy the process immensely.* **Two,** *slowly, gently, normal sensation returning to your body and you may wiggle your fingers and your toes and* **One,** *returning to full conscious awareness, aware again of the sounds in the room and eyes open wide, wide, wide awake feeling absolutely marvelous. If you like, give yourself a positive mental suggestion as you reorient back to the room.*

7 Radiation

Before you begin, get comfortable, make sure that your neck and head are supported, then settle back and find a spot on the ceiling that you can focus on. The spot should be just above your forehead so that it causes a slight strain on the eyes as they focus upwards. Once you have your eyes fixated on that spot on the ceiling do not move your head or your gaze anywhere else, and just begin to count slowly from 1-5.

One, ... *focus on your breathing... and allow your breathing to slow down and relax .... Take a nice deep breath in... hold it... and then exhale slowly and notice how comfortable it feels. You are supported so you can just let go and relax.* **Two,** *... as you continue staring at the spot on the ceiling you might find that after a while it may begin to distort, go fuzzy, or move around a little and that's just fine, whatever happens is meant to happen.* **Three,** *... listen to all of the sounds around you, these sounds are unimportant, discard them and whatever you hear from* *now on will only help to relax you even more . And as you continue staring at that spot on the ceiling notice how tired your eyes are beginning to feel. The eyelids are becoming heavier and heavier, droopy and drowsy, drowsy and droopy, so heavy, so relaxed and you may notice that they begin to blink more frequently as you relax even deeper.* **Four,** *... imagine for a moment that the air you are breathing in has a deeply tranquilizing quality to it and each and every time you inhale you slip deeper and deeper into comfort and trance. And as you continue to breathe slowly and deeply and to stare at that spot on the ceiling notice that your eyes are beginning to tear up just a little bit and you are looking forward to closing those heavy eyelids and relaxing... and...* **Five,** *... close those heavy eyelids and feel a wave of relaxation move through your body, from the top of your head to the tips of your toes, as you enter into that inner world, that lovely peaceful place we call trance. For a while you find yourself just floating and drifting, drifting and floating on a sea of dreams with nothing to worry about, no one to please and nothing to do except relax. You're allowing the trance to deepen by itself, removing yourself from daily concerns and simply enjoying your own time. Relaxing, releasing, letting go as you drift down and down into a wonderful hypnotic sleep.*

When you begin your first radiation treatment you will feel a deep sense of peace, serenity and tranquility moving gently through your body relaxing and releasing all stresses and concerns. You know that the radiation will help to destroy the cancer cells in your body. The rays are your friends and can clear the body of unwelcome invaders and allow it to return to a state of balance and harmony. These rays are strong and direct and their aim is perfect, they make a direct hit on the cancer cells in your body and they destroy them completely, completely. Meanwhile you can surround your healthy cells with a protective coat that is impenetrable to the radiation. Decide which color this coating is perhaps it is a bright vibrant color or maybe a soft pastel shade... is it thick or is it fine, yet strong? Imagine it in your mind's eye as you continue to relax deeper and deeper. The noise that the machine makes will remind you of a period in your life when you felt wonderfully relaxed. Perhaps it was an occasion you spent with a good friend or friends, or a time out in nature when you savored the sights and sounds of the natural environment. It really doesn't matter which memory comes to mind as long as it is relaxing. To your surprise the time you spend receiving the radiation will seem to pass very quickly and it will be easy for you to remain motionless, so wonderfully easy. Once the treatment is finished imagine applying a healing ointment over your skin, which moisturizes the skin cells and keeps them supple and healthy. Know also that your own inner resources will continue to heal and strengthen your body.

Now enjoy your special place for a few moments longer then I am going to count from 5 down to 1 and when I reach the number 1 you will come back to full conscious awareness feeling very, very good. **Five***, you have done some good work today and you are learning how to use the power of your subconscious mind to help and heal yourself.* **Four,** *each and every time you choose to do this kind of therapy, whether with me or another hypnotherapist or listening to your recording you will go deeper and faster than the time before.* **Three,** *you will gain great healing benefits and enjoy the process immensely.* **Two,** *slowly, gently, normal sensation returning to your body and you may wiggle your fingers and your toes and* **One,** *returning to full conscious awareness, aware again of the sounds in the room and eyes open wide, wide, wide awake feeling absolutely marvelous. If you like, give yourself a positive mental suggestion as you reorient back to the room.*

8 Pain.

In the following, it's important to exhale slowly and only add the odd number when you are ready to inhale. When the word sleep is used in the following trance it does not mean fall asleep it simply means allow your body to relax completely.

*Start by making yourself comfortable, sitting or lying down **(remember not to lie flat as you may unwittingly fall asleep)**, your head and neck supported with cushions or pillows. I am going to count upwards and as I do so I want you to open your eyes and inhale on the odd numbers and close them and exhale on the even numbers just like a slow blink. Each time you close your eyes you will become more and more relaxed until eventually you will be so relaxed that it will be almost impossible to open those weary eyelids. When they finally remain shut you will be in a deep state of hypnosis. So let's begin **1**, take a nice deep breath, open those eyes and each time you open the eyes, focus on the tip of your nose. **2**, close those eyes and exhale slowly, letting the air all the way out, good. **3**, inhale and open the eyes. **4**, close the eyes and release all the tension and stresses of the day as you exhale slowly, so good to relax and to let go. **5**, open the eyes and notice that it's becoming more difficult to do so. **6**, close them and feel a deep sense of peace move through your body from the top of your head to the tips of your toes, and as you exhale your eyelids begin to feel heavier and heavier **7**, open those weary eyes and **8**, close them and slip deeper and deeper into comfort and trance, nothing to worry about and nothing to do except let yourself relax. **9**, open those eyes if they are able and **10**, close them and notice that it is becoming almost impossible for you to open them, it feels as if those eyelids are stuck together and it is just too much effort to move them. **11**, open and **12**, close those eyes and sink deeper and deeper into peace and tranquility as if you are floating* *on a sea of dreams. Floating and drifting, drifting and floating deeper, deeper, deeper, relaxed.(You can go on counting as long or as briefly as is necessary until your eyelids stay firmly shut)*

Become aware of the way your body is feeling. Imagine a light slowly passing down through your body from the top of your head to the tips of your toes, like a scanner able to detect areas of tension. Whenever that light hits on any tension in your body it is able to magically dissolve that tension, see it disappear or feel it simply melt away. Flowing down like molten candle wax, down, down, down into a deep hypnotic sleep. Notice as your body relaxes, the feeling of the air against your face and as you notice this you slip deeper and deeper into sleep. Now become aware of the feeling of your clothes against your skin and slip even deeper still. And finally become aware of the feeling of the sofa (bed etc) pushing up against your back and relax even more into a deep hypnotic sleep.

If you are suffering from persistent or periodical pain you can learn how to reduce that pain to a comfortable level. Begin by imagining that you are an artist standing in front of a large, life-sized sheet of canvas, propped up on an easel. By your side is a palette with different colors of paint and various paintbrushes. In the background your favorite piece of music is playing and the notes help you to relax more and more deeply. You gently run your fingers over the surface of the canvas, feeling it's texture, soothing and reassuring. Lifting up one of the brushes you run the bristle head down across your palm, creating a pleasant sensation.

Now you are ready to begin and dipping the brush into the paint you boldly draw a life-size outline of your body. *And every thought, every sound, every sensation takes you deeper and deeper into comfort and sleep.*

Next, focus on the areas of pain in your body, locate their exact position, one by one, by slowly scanning through the body starting at the top of the head and carefully moving gently down to the tips of the toes.

Whenever an area of discomfort is located, stop and spend time examining the area, if it has a color what color would that be ... is it large or small... does it have a shape ... does it radiate outwards or is it focused only on one area?

Now listen for the sound it makes, is the pitch high or low? What does it feel like, does it throb, or is the sensation sharp or dull? If you could rate the pain on a scale of 1-10 with 10 being the most intense it can be where does it fall on that scale? Take your time and really experience the pain and then begin to change it. *And every thought, every sound, every sensation takes you deeper and deeper into comfort and sleep.*

Take the paintbrush and paint the pain onto the canvas, move it out of your body, transfer it to the canvas. If the pain is in your head place it in the same area on the canvas, and as you do this feel the discomfort diminish. Paint every detail, the intensity of it, the color, shape, size and sound of it and as you do so, relief gently permeates that part of your body. Slowly at first and then more quickly as you relax even deeper enjoying this increase in comfort. It is as if the paint forms a liquid arch from the body to the canvas and the pain gently flows over to the cloth. And as it flows out of the body, a little at first and then more and more, the discomfort diminishes and is replaced with feelings of comfort. *And every thought, every sound, every sensation takes you deeper and deeper into comfort and sleep.*

Now take the paintbrush and lighten the color of the pain on the canvas by adding a healing color and surprisingly you begin to feel even more relief. Continue to do this with all uncomfortable areas in your body taking as long as you need until you feel much more at ease.

Now enjoy your special place for a few moments longer then I am going to count from 5 down to 1 and when I reach the number 1 you will come back to full conscious awareness feeling very, very good. **Five,** *you have done some good work today and you are learning how to use the power of your subconscious mind to help and heal yourself.* **Four,** *each and every time you choose to do this kind of therapy, whether with me or another hypnotherapist or listening to your recording you will go deeper and faster than the time before.* **Three,** *you will gain great healing benefits and enjoy the process immensely.* **Two,** *slowly, gently, normal sensation returning to your body and you may wiggle your fingers and your toes and* **One,** *returning to full conscious awareness, aware again of the sounds in the room and eyes open wide, wide, wide awake feeling absolutely marvelous. If you like you can give yourself a positive mental suggestion as you reorient back to the room.*

9 Nausea.

Take a nice deep breath, close your eyes and relax. Imagine that you're watching a feather as it moves slowly down towards the earth. Your eyes are fixated on that feather and you take another slow deep breath and as you exhale, begin counting how long it takes before the feather comes to rest on a soft, mossy embankment. **1,** *as you count you find your whole body beginning to relax more and more. It's almost as if you are floating on the feather. Gliding downwards, safely, gently, softly, into relaxation and even the count itself takes you deeper still.* **2,** *letting go still more. The feather is white and fluffy, medium sized and you wonder what kind of a bird it belonged to and where that bird is now.* **3,** *deeper, deeper, deeper, relaxed. In your* mind you may hear a beautiful melody that accompanies the downward motion of the feather, soothing you like a gentle massage. Easing away all the tensions of the day, the notes in perfect harmony. **4,** letting go still more. You might enjoy the physical sensations of floating slowly downwards, a gentle breeze brushing against your cheeks, the warmth of the sun on your body and the softness of the feather underfoot. **5,** deeper, deeper, deeper, relaxed. You wonder what it would be like if you had the ability to fly, to soar on the wind, free like a bird. **6,** letting go still more. The different scents and fragrances, subtle yet distinct, reach your nostrils, the perfume of summer blossoms reminds you of happy memories and it seems that you are floating on a sea of dreams. **7,** deeper, deeper, deeper, relaxed. Floating and drifting, drifting and floating, so comfortable, so secure as if you are enveloped by a warm blanket of tranquility. **8,** letting go still more. The sky is that wonderful shade of blue that you find particularly relaxing and there are occasional white, fluffy clouds floating past and melodic birdsong in the distance. **9,** deeper, deeper, deeper, relaxed. Your feather is almost ready to land on a patch of soft, green, mossy earth. When it does, you can enjoy this special place for 2 minutes of clock time, all the time in hypnosis time that you will need to slip deeper and deeper into trance. To the level of trance, which is just right for you today. I will not tell you what to do during that time, you might decide to sit back and relax or go exploring and whatever you decide it will be very enjoyable and extremely relaxing. **10,** your feather has landed- enjoy the sights, sounds, aromas and sensations of your mossy embankment.

Pause for 2 minutes

We all enjoy reminiscing from time to time with memories from childhood, from our teenage years and later on into adulthood. Perhaps you remember in school, in chemistry class the first time the teacher took a beaker of bubbling liquid. He added something to it and lo and behold like magic the bubbling stopped and the liquid in the beaker became calm and serene. Miraculous in a sense and although you didn't quite understand how it worked the transformation was impressive.

Or, perhaps you remember the first time swimming in a pool, sea, lake or river when you put your head under the water and looked beneath the surface. On top you could hear the noises of people laughing and talking but underneath the surface, all was quiet and peaceful.

Maybe you remember your mother's gentle embrace when you felt unwell, her soothing touch upon your brow, a warm hot water bottle to hold next to your stomach and the stories she told, filling you with awe and wonder. Princesses and dragons, knights and damsels in distress, a world where all is possible and you began to feel better, being loved and cared for.

Perhaps she told you the story of the magic pill, a small, round pill, easy to swallow with a clean and pleasant taste. When you swallow this pill everything inside feels better, as if the storm, which has been raging, subsides, everything settling down, calm, peaceful and relaxed, your whole body responding to this tiny magic pill feeling better and better.

Now enjoy your special place for a few moments longer then I am going to count from 5 down to 1 and when I reach the number 1 you will come back to full conscious awareness feeling very, very good. **Five**, *you have done some good work today and you are learning how to use the power of your subconscious mind to help and heal yourself.* **Four,** *each and every time you choose to do this kind of therapy, whether with me or another hypnotherapist or listening to your recording you will go deeper and faster than the time before.* **Three,** *you will gain great healing* benefits and enjoy the process immensely. **Two,** *slowly, gently, normal sensation returning to your body and you may wiggle your fingers and your toes and* **One,** *returning to full conscious awareness, aware again of the sounds in the room and eyes open wide, wide, wide awake feeling absolutely marvelous. If you like you can give yourself a positive mental suggestion as you reorient back to the room.*

10 Tumor Reduction

This induction may be used before, after or in conjunction with treatment.

Before you begin make sure your clothing is loose and relaxed. Take a nice, slow, deep breath, close your eyes and as the air slowly fills your lungs settle back comfortably. Notice the feeling as the air enters your nostrils and as you exhale allow the breath to exit through your nose in order to slow down the entire process. When you are ready take in another breath, focus on the feeling of the air travelling through your nose, down your throat and into your lungs and feel the expansion of your lungs. Really become aware of the mechanism of your breathing. Now I'd like you to continue breathing deeply and slowly, noticing as you do how relaxed your body is beginning to feel. Nothing to worry about, nothing to do, this is your time to just enjoy the rest and breathe deeply. I will be quiet for one minute of clock time to allow you to continue breathing slowly and relaxedly.

... **Pause for one minute** ...

Now imagine that it is fall. You are inside a cozy log cabin sitting in a rocking chair by a roaring fire, which casts a rosy glow about the room. The logs crackle as they burn and there is the fresh smell of burning wood as you rock back and forth, back and forth, back and forth. There's a soft warm blanket draped over your shoulders, and you feel peaceful and tranquil.

The cabin is surrounded by trees and you look out of the window and upwards at the autumn canopy above you. Most of the leaves are red and gold and they dance above your head as the wind whistles through them. You can hear the wind as it rattles against the window panes. You pull your warm blanket closer to your body and snuggle into it. Dreamily you watch some of the leaves detach from the stems and twirl delicately down and down before coming to rest and curtseying on the soft earth below. You imagine how it would feel if you ventured outside. The autumn wind cool on your cheek, refreshing, ruffling your hair and swirling around you.

You imagine picking up a freshly fallen leaf and rubbing it gently between your fingers, the texture somehow comforting. And later the joy of crunching over the drier, older, copper colored leaves beneath your feet as you run through them.

But you are not outside, you are warm and relaxed inside and you can watch the sudden gusts of wind lift up the swirling leaves, moving them continuously around and around, around and around, around and around. You sit in your rocking chair, sipping hot chocolate and rock back and forth, back and forth, back and forth as the leaves fall down and down and you go deeper and deeper relaxed.

Now from this place of deep relaxation imagine what your immune system might look like, create the imagery. Perhaps you see it as a pack of English bulldogs, ferocious and strong, marching through your body, symbolizing the strength and protectiveness of your immune system.

Imagine these English bulldogs snarling, growling, and biting into the tumor and devouring it. See the tumor diminish in size as the cancer cells are killed and completely consumed by the dogs. Watch the tumor as it shrinks down and down, smaller and smaller and watch the white blood cells clear up any debris so that it can be safely eliminated through your feces and urine. The weak cancer cells are destroyed, eradicated, annihilated and the tumor continues to diminish in size until it disappears…

You feel a healing occurring within your body and you know that your health is being restored.

The power of the mind is incredible as is the body's ability to heal itself. Each time you listen to this recording the power of these healing suggestions will be magnified 10 times and take complete and thorough effect upon your mind, body and spirit.

Now enjoy your special place for a few moments longer then I am going to count from 5 down to 1 and when I reach the number 1 you will come back to full conscious awareness feeling very, very good. **Five**, *you have done some good work today and you are learning how to use the power of your subconscious mind to help and heal yourself.* **Four,** *each and every time you choose to do this kind of therapy, whether with me or another hypnotherapist or listening to your recording you will go deeper and faster than the time before.* **Three,** *you will gain great healing benefits and enjoy the process immensely.* **Two,** *slowly, gently, normal sensation returning to your body and you may wiggle your fingers and your toes and* **One,** *returning to full conscious awareness, aware again of the sounds in the room and eyes open wide, wide, wide awake feeling absolutely marvelous. If you like you can give yourself a positive mental suggestion as you reorient back to the room.*

9: Inductions for Healing:

Depending on the types of treatment we decide upon recovery from breast cancer may be a slow process and the desire to return to normal healthy functioning is strong. We long to be able to do the things we did pre-cancer whether it be working, travelling, caring for our families, socializing or enjoying recreational pursuits. To accelerate healing the following inductions may be used and it's important to remember that the more you practice hypnosis the better you become at it and the more effective it will be.

11 Healing Induction Using The Coin Drop

Before using this induction make sure you are sitting upright with your head and neck supported. This is important because occasionally as relaxation occurs the neck may fall to one side. Next put a coin between your thumb and index finger and hold your arm out in front of you, with your wrist facing downwards.

Now focus all of your attention on your thumbnail and don't let your gaze move. As you do so you begin to notice how heavy the coin is beginning to feel. Notice also the different sensation in the tips of the fingers, they might feel hot or cool, heavy or light, tingly or tremulous. As you continue to focus on the nail the eyelids become heavier and heavier and your eyes may begin to water just a little at first. Eventually they close and then you can imagine a wave of relaxation moving through your body. Slowly the coin begins to feel even heavier and eventually it slips gently through your fingers and falls to the ground below.

When the coin hits the floor that is a signal to your subconscious mind to enter trance and to allow a second wave of relaxation to pass through your body. Now your arm feels heavy and tired and you can slowly move that arm down towards your lap and as it touches your lap you can go twice as deep as you were before.

*Next I'd like you to take 5 slow, deep breaths and with each exhalation you find yourself drifting deeper and deeper into comfort and trance until after the fifth breath you are very deeply relaxed. **1,** inhale slowly, filling your lungs with air, hold this... and as you exhale release all the stress and tension and slip deeper and deeper into relaxation. **2,** inhale deeply, hold the air... and as you release feel yourself sinking down and down, more and more into a state of quiet tranquility. **3,** take a deep breath in, hold it... and as you breathe out blow away all the worries and cares of the day. **4,** inhale deeply, hold the air... and as you exhale go deeper and deeper relaxed and **5,** inhale, hold the air... and as you let it escape feel yourself move all the way down, all the way down into a very peaceful state of relaxation.*

Imagine that it's a warm summer's day, not too hot just right and you are out walking along the bank of a beautiful river enjoying nature.

The geese and ducks are the only visible inhabitants on the river and there's the occasional splash of a fish as it surfaces through the water in search of food. The path you are on is deserted except for an old man sitting a distance ahead on a bench. As you approach he smiles and the two of you begin to exchange pleasantries. Through the course of the conversation he tells you that he is a healer. He says you too are in need of healing and you nod in agreement surprised that he is aware of your plight.

He tells you he can help and all you have to do is follow his guidance so you sit down on the grassy verge and listen to his words. The old man tells you to close your eyes and imagine a warm golden ball in the centre of your body, soft yet vibrant, filled with healing energy. Using your inner eye, watch as it slowly begins to radiate outwards all through your body and soon you can even feel its soft warmth as it gently bathes your cells in its golden light. You bask in the knowledge that the light is healing and cleansing every cell, every tissue, every organ of your body. And the golden ball is accompanied with music, at first, barely audible but gradually as the light expands the music becomes more distinct and a beautiful melody bursts forth travelling through your body and lifting you to great heights.

It seems as if you are becoming lighter and lighter as if you are floating higher and higher, up on a cloud, high above all the cares and concerns of the day. Around you, is the faintest fragrance, a scent, which is pleasing and familiar, soothing you, reminding you of happy times. Now your body is glowing with golden light and the healing intensifies. The old man tells you to open your eyes and look at your reflection in the river. As you gaze into the waters you see yourself transformed, all systems in your body are working maximally, your cells, organs and tissues are healthy and this renewed vitality creates joy. You are able once more to move with ease and agility, doing all the things you love to do.

The old man smiles at you, he says he must leave but now he has shown you the way and all you have to do is practice this manifestation every day and good health will be yours. You thank him and watch as he walks off into the distance, safe in the knowledge that this transformation is taking place.

Now enjoy your special place for a few moments longer then I am going to count from 5 down to 1 and when I reach the number 1 you will come back to full conscious awareness feeling very, very good. **Five**, *you have done some good work today and you are learning how to use the power of your subconscious mind to help and heal yourself.* **Four,** *each and every time you choose to do this kind of therapy, whether with me or another hypnotherapist or listening to your recording you will go deeper and faster than the time before.* **Three,** *you will gain great healing benefits and enjoy the process immensely.* **Two,** *slowly, gently, normal sensation returning to your body and you may wiggle your fingers and your toes and* **One,** *returning to full conscious awareness, aware again of the sounds in the room and eyes open, wide, wide awake feeling absolutely marvelous. If you like you can give yourself a positive mental suggestion as you reorient back to the room.*

12 The Fairystory.

Note. I am using a meadow as a safe place but you may substitute this with your safe place, which can be anywhere you choose, a beach, a forest, or your own home. Just remember to bring the scene to life by detailing what you might see, smell, taste, hear or touch in your safe place.

Imagine a meadow on a beautiful spring day. The grass so green and fresh, the wild flowers dotted around as if an artist has haphazardly splashed small bursts of color here and there. The young lambs are frolicking about, happy to be alive. Bordering the meadow are a few scattered trees, standing tall and proud with their budding leaves beginning to open and a small brook running alongside the edge.

Listen to the birds singing, familiar, comforting, joyous and watch as the wind skittles across the grass creating a wave like motion. Feel the air brush gently across your cheek. Hear the water as it travels over stones and pebbles on its way to the far distant ocean. Look at the sunlight falling over the meadow creating different patterns of shade and light depending on the cloud formation. It's a beautiful peaceful, spring day and you feel safe and at peace with the world.

As you meander through the meadow you notice an incline on the west side so you make your way over and see 10 wooden steps leading to a field down below, which has a tiny cottage in the middle. Intrigued you decide to make your way down to the cottage and as you take each step down you drift deeper and deeper into comfort and trance and even the count itself will take you deeper still. **1,** *... you notice smoke coming from the cottage chimney.* **2,** *... deeper, deeper, deeper relaxed.* **3,** *you can smell the burning wood.* **4,** *... deeper, deeper relaxed.* **5,** *the steps beneath you feel sturdy and strong as does the wooden handrail you are holding.* **6,** *... letting go still more.* **7,** *an old woman comes out of the cottage, she notices you, and waving, shouts: "Hello."* **8,** *... deeper, deeper, deeper relaxed.* **9,** *she beckons you over... and* **10,** *at the bottom of the staircase deeply, deeply, relaxed.*

You walk over to the old woman and she tells you she is a storyteller and that she has a special story just for you. Delighted you sit down alongside the old woman and listen as she begins her tale. The words and her voice hold you spellbound and you continue to drift deeper and deeper into comfort and trance.

'Once upon a time there was a princess who became very ill. The best physicians in the court were called in to diagnose the princess's ailment and after they had done so they treated her and waited expectantly for a healthy transformation to occur. None however was forthcoming for although they had removed the problem the princess failed to thrive… **Deeper, deeper relaxed, deeper with every breath you exhale.**

The physicians scratched their heads in bewilderment and so in desperation the king called the court magician and asked him what could be done to help his daughter. The magician pondered the question and then asked that he meet with the princess to assess her condition. The king agreed and the magician met with the young princess who indeed looked very frail. He asked her, "Are you eating properly?" to which the princess replied sadly, "No." Then he asked, "Are you exercising?" and again she replied "No." "What do you do all day?" asked the magician. "After the physicians treated me I felt so weak that I don't do much of anything, I just lie in bed most of the day feeling sad." she replied… And every **thought, every sound, every sensation takes you deeper still.**

"Come over here," beckoned the magician "and look in this full length mirror. What do you see?" The princess looked woefully at her reflection, she appeared pale and gaunt…"I look terrible." she sighed. "Yes," said the magician, "but this is not a true reflection, none of the mirrors in your kingdom will show you the true, healthy, vibrant you." The princess looked surprised and the magician continued, "Out there somewhere over the hills and dales there is a magic apple tree and besides it is a mirror. When you bite the magic apple and swallow it you will again be well and the mirrors reflection will show you your true reflection, healthy and vibrant… **Deeper, deeper relaxed with every breath you exhale.**

Until that time all the mirrors in the kingdom shall be covered and in order to find this tree and mirror you must search for them on foot. It is only you who can find them however a lady in waiting may accompany you on these walks. "But I am so weak." said the princess. "Yes that's true", said the magician, "so you must begin slowly by eating a little and walking a little, and that way you will eventually be able to find the magic fruit."

The princess really wanted to find that fruit so in order to gain enough strength for the quest she began to eat a little food and to walk a little each day. At first she could not venture far and her search was limited but as the days passed into weeks and then months the princess's appetite increased and she walked further and further. At the beginning the process was very difficult and painful, her muscles ached and it was hard to eat any food but slowly bit-by-bit, she began to feel better and her body ached less and less. In fact the princess enjoyed the beauty of the outdoors. She was driven, she had a purpose and she was determined to find that magic fruit tree ... **And every thought, every sound, every sensation takes you deeper still.**

A year passed by and one day on her sojourns, the princess came across an apple tree beside which stood the magician. Next to him was a full-length mirror. "Is this it?" asked the princess excitedly. "Yes." replied the magician with delight. "Here take a bite of this lovely apple." The princess did so, it tasted juicy and sweet and she swallowed the fruit quickly. "Now look in the mirror," said the magician. The princess did as she was told and there in front of her stood a healthy young woman, vibrant and strong. "I am well again!" she exclaimed. "Yes," replied the magician, "and now all the mirrors in the kingdom can be uncovered as they will all reflect your true health and beauty." The king and the courtiers rejoiced and there was great celebration in the kingdom as their princess was once again healthy and strong.'

The old woman smiles as she finishes the story and you thank her and take your leave climbing back up the staircase to the meadow above, pondering her words.

Now enjoy your special place for a few moments longer then I am going to count from 5 down to 1 and when I reach the number 1 you will come back to full conscious awareness feeling very, very good. **Five**, *you have done some good work today and you are learning how to use the power of your subconscious mind to help and heal yourself.* **Four,** *each and every time you choose to do this kind of therapy, whether with me or another hypnotherapist or listening to your recording you will go deeper and faster than the time before.* **Three,** *you will gain great healing benefits and enjoy the process immensely.* **Two,** *slowly, gently, normal sensation returning to your body and you may wiggle your fingers and your toes and* **One,** *returning to full conscious awareness, aware again of the sounds in the room and eyes open wide, wide awake feeling absolutely marvelous. If you like you can give yourself a positive mental suggestion as you reorient back to the room.*

13 Dream Lake (Relaxation Induction)

Sit down in a comfortable chair, with your head and neck supported and take a nice deep breath, inhaling through your nose for the count of 4... holding the air for 4 seconds... and exhaling slowly through your nose ... Imagine that you are breathing in peace and tranquility and breathing out stress and tension. Do this again, slowly inhaling ... holding the breath ... and slowly exhaling through the nose... Notice how comfortable your body is beginning to feel. And again inhale... hold... and exhale... With each exhalation you become more and more relaxed. Finally one more deep breath inwards.... hold the air for 4 seconds... and as you release it feel your body move even deeper into comfort and relaxation.

Now imagine your favorite color starting as a wave of relaxation at the top of your head and slowly moving down through your body to the tips of your toes.

As it moves down it touches and relaxes every part of your body and the more relaxed you become the better you feel. All of the muscles in the scalp and neck begin to relax as that beautiful color touches them and as the color moves down over the face all of those muscles begin to relax and let go. The forehead smooths out and relaxes and even the tiny muscles around the eyes, the nose and the mouth release and let go. And as this happens you move deeper and deeper into comfort and trance.

Now that beautiful color moves along the shoulders and into each of your arms. See the bicep muscles tight, taut and tense and the moment that color touches them they let go and relax. Then the color moves down through the elbows and around the elbows and into the muscles of the forearms and these muscles let go and relax and you go deeper and deeper into comfort and trance. Then the color moves into your hands and out through your fingertips so now you have a wave of relaxation moving from the top of your head, across your shoulders, down both arms and out through your fingertips.

Take another nice deep breath, as the color moves into your chest and your stomach relaxing all the muscles there. And at the same time imagine a wave of relaxation moving down your back, down, down, down, to the lower part of your back. These muscles let go and with every breath you exhale you slip deeper and deeper into comfort and trance.

The beautiful color continues to move downwards through your hips and yours thighs and notice what it feels like for the thigh muscles to let go and relax. The color moves down each leg around the knees and through the knees and into the calf muscles. And again imagine these tight, taut and tense and the moment that color touches them they release and let go.

Now the beautiful color moves into the feet and out through the toes and it is as if the feet have been tightly bound and the moment the color touches them they are able to spread out and relax. And your whole body is deeply relaxed as this wave of relaxation washes over and through you from the top of your head to the tips of your toes.

Imagine lying in a hammock on a hot sunny day rocking back and forth, back and forth, back and forth until the rocking lulls you into a deep and peaceful sleep. And as you sleep you have a dream. You dream that you are transported to the side of a huge lake but this is no ordinary lake it is a dream lake.

Sunlight dances along the surface of the water and there are patches of vibrant color, beautiful blues, vivid violet and emerald green. The colors look like bright oil paints and they appear to have depth and texture so that it seems as if the crests of the waves are thick and frothy. Shrubbery surrounds the lake, the land is flat by the water's edge then slowly rises from the valley floor to form gently sloping hills. The lily pads on the water's surface have texture and depth and as you stretch out to touch them they move towards you and follow the motion of your hand. Surprised you tentatively touch the surface of the water and it too follows the motion of your hand. As you are doing this you think of the last time you swam in a lake and instantaneously the image of this memory appears in front of you. Could it be that the movement of your hand coincides with your thoughts to create whatever you imagine?

Gingerly you touch the water again and think of your last picnic and lo and behold it forms in front of you. How wonderful. Suddenly you remember how easy it was to create an imaginary world when you were a child and you feel that childish wonder once more.

Your one wish is to be well, to feel healthy and comfortable in your body, pain free and strong. You touch the waters again and think of spiritual/religious leaders from history, Jesus, Buddha, Mother Theresa or some other healers and watch closely as one of these individuals manifests before your eyes. Watch as he/she moves towards you. Notice what he/ she is wearing. Notice every feature, every mannerism. Listen as this individual bids you welcome in a resonating voice, which is strangely calming and has a different cadence. He/she stretches out his/her hands to you and as you place your hands in his/hers you feel a deep connection. Look into his/her eyes and as you do all discomfort vanishes, there is only peace and understanding an indescribable familiarity. You are safe. Mentally ask to be healed and feel that healing begin … you are being transformed.

Pause for 2 minutes.

Eventually the healer releases his/her hold and as he/she moves away your eyes lock one last time. You both smile at each other and you telepathically thank him/her, then your healer disappears. Your body feels different, you feel different, a healing has taken place and you know that you can visit your healer again whenever you want to.

Now enjoy your special place for a few moments longer then I am going to count from 5 down to 1 and when I

reach the number 1 you will come back to full conscious awareness feeling very, very good. **Five,** *you have done some good work today and you are learning how to use the power of your subconscious mind to help and heal yourself.* **Four,** *each and every time you choose to do this kind of therapy, whether with me or another hypnotherapist or listening to your recording you will go deeper and faster than the time before.* **Three,** *you will gain great healing benefits and enjoy the process immensely.* **Two,** *slowly, gently, normal sensation returning to your body and you may wiggle your fingers and your toes and* **One,** *returning to full conscious awareness, aware again of the sounds in the room and eyes open wide, wide awake feeling absolutely marvelous. If you like you can give yourself a positive mental suggestion as you reorient back to the room.*

By now you will probably have developed a preference for one or two introductory inductions, which suit you and enable you to enter trance easily. These are the italicized paragraphs at the beginning of each script. Whether it's a progressive muscle relaxation, the coin drop, eye fixation, imagery or one of the others doesn't matter as long as it appeals to you. To make the remaining scripts even more effective you may now select your favorite italicized induction and preface the suggestions that follow.

14 The Spa

Imagine a day at the spa, a day of luxurious pampering and deep relaxation. Changing into a swimsuit and donning a soft white robe and slippers you make your way outdoors to the naturally occurring waters of the spa. Steam rises gently from the surface of the waters and there's a faint smell of mineral salts. A tall leafy green tree offers shade from the hot sun, its leaves waxily shining in the light. **And the**

warm gentle breeze lulls you deeper and deeper into comfort and trance.

Surreptitiously you dip your toe in the water, it feels soothingly warm and comfortable and you slowly lower half of your body into the bubbling liquid. Almost at once the bubbles massage your limbs, easing away all aches and pains and you submerge yourself up to your shoulders. It's so relaxing, so comfortable like a thousand tiny hands massaging and caressing your body. Suddenly in the middle of this summer's day an unexpected cloud gives way to a rain shower just above you and large cool raindrops fall on your head and shoulders, contrasting beautifully with the balmy waters of the spa. **And the warm gentle breeze lulls you deeper and deeper into comfort and trance.**

While relaxing you drift and dream and dream and drift, imagining what a spa might be like in Roman Times at a banquet on midsummer's eve. Their pool, open to the starry night sky has large, white, fluted pillars towering upwards from the corners of the structure and statutes adorning the terrace. Swimmers immerse themselves in the healing waters while men and women dressed in tunics and Togas slowly, majestically make their way towards the banquet. A veritable feast is laid out before them. **And the warm gentle breeze lulls you deeper and deeper into comfort and trance.**

Soothed by these images you realize it's time to leave the waters and go for a facial and a full body massage. How lovely to feel the cool moist creams being gently eased over your face, then cleansed with a hot steamy cloth, sensations of heat and coolness, coolness and heat, pleasant, relaxing.

And oh the joy of those essential oils covering the body, releasing, relaxing and letting go. The fragrances, the sense of touch, feathery and light, followed by deep heavy pressure then lightness, lightness and pressure and the soft sound of sensual music. As your breathing slows down even more, there's nothing to do, no one to please, just let yourself be. **And the warm gentle breeze lulls you deeper and deeper into comfort and trance.**

Finally completely destressed you lie in the recovery room, simply being, every muscle, every tissue, every cell of your body so deeply relaxed. And as you relax you have a dream, a dream that the healing waters of the spa have reenergized and restored you and you feel yourself vibrant, enthusiastic and powerful once again. **And these feelings stay with you and grow stronger as you continue to get better and better.**

Now enjoy your special place for a few moments longer then I am going to count from 5 down to 1 and when I reach the number 1 you will come back to full conscious awareness feeling very, very good. ***Five****, you have done some good work today and you are learning how to use the power of your subconscious mind to help and heal yourself.* ***Four****, each and every time you choose to do this kind of therapy, whether with me or another hypnotherapist or listening to your recording you will go deeper and faster than the time before.* ***Three****, you will gain great healing benefits and enjoy the process immensely.* ***Two****, slowly, gently, normal sensation returning to your body and you may wiggle your fingers and your toes and* ***One****, returning to full conscious awareness, aware again of the sounds in the room and eyes open, wide, wide awake feeling absolutely marvelous. If you like you can give yourself a positive mental suggestion as you reorient back to the room.*

15 Simple Things

As before you may select an introductory, italicized, induction of your choice to preface the following suggestions.

Focus on your breathing and take slow, deep, rhythmic breaths, noticing the difference between each and every inhalation and each and every exhalation. While you are drifting let your mind float as light as a feather, as light as bubbles drifting through the air. Bubbles, round, smooth, magical... see the wonder and joy on children's faces when they blow bubbles. A simple thing made out of soapy water that can give such pleasure to the young and sometimes not so young. Wet to the touch, transparent and when you look closely often colorful. So many simple things that give us pleasure each day. **And your breathing slows and your mind drifts as you slip deeper and deeper into hypnosis.**

A woman once told me she loved stretching her arms and legs in bed when she wakened up each morning, the warmth of the sheets against her body, the joy of wakening slowly. She said that first cup of tea in the morning, the hot reassuring liquid slipping down her throat as she cupped her hands around her favorite mug was pleasantly familiar. Reassuring, something she had done most of her life. **And your breathing slows and your mind drifts as you slip deeper and deeper into hypnosis.**

Switching the radio on and listening to the music as she prepared for the day ahead. Morning rituals, so different for everyone... and within each, simple pleasures go unnoticed ... The feeling of a hot shower on a cold morning can be comforting, while some find pleasure in a cold, refreshing shower and others enjoy the warm, hot steamy relaxation of a bath. The fragrance of bath oils or a bubble bath, the soothing warmth, the silkiness of the oils against the skin, a slow and leisurely stretch are all simple pleasures. **And your breathing slows and your mind drifts as you slip deeper and deeper into hypnosis.**

Watching a favorite TV show or becoming immersed in a great book, reality put on pause, while the mind soars with possibilities, no barriers, no boundaries… Baking, the joy of kneading dough, the feel of the dough under your hands, the smell as it rises in the oven and the delight in eating freshly baked bread … Being in the garden, that oasis of peace, colorful, scented, tranquil, with only the sound of birdsong and the buzzing of the bees. The joy of watching a hummingbird hover by a flower as it feeds on the nectar.

Simple pleasures, so many of them in a day, so many go unnoticed. What did you enjoy today?

Pause for 2 minutes

Now relax in your special place for a few moments longer then I am going to count from 5 down to 1 and when I reach the number 1 you will come back to full conscious awareness feeling very, very good. **Five,** *you have done some good work today and you are learning how to use the power of your subconscious mind to help and heal yourself.* **Four,** *each and every time you choose to do this kind of therapy, whether with me or another hypnotherapist or listening to your recording you will go deeper and faster than the time before.* **Three,** *you will gain great healing benefits and enjoy the process immensely.* **Two,** *slowly, gently, normal sensation returning to your body and you may wiggle your fingers and your toes and* **One,** *returning to full conscious awareness, aware again of the sounds in the room and eyes open wide, wide awake feeling absolutely marvelous. If you like you can give yourself a positive mental suggestion as you reorient back to the room.*

10: Inductions to Cope with Depression

Depression is common amongst cancer patients. The shock of receiving a life threatening diagnosis is in itself traumatic and the fear and anxiety around treatment and an uncertain future makes us more susceptible to this mood disorder. Depression may occur at any time, shortly after diagnosis, throughout treatment or recovery and even years later when a person is deemed cancer-free. There are many reasons for this, changes in our bodies, energy levels, work and relationships, which may all negatively affect us. The inductions below are designed to help elevate mood and may be used alone as you travel through your cancer journey. But if your depression symptoms are extreme it is essential to talk to your doctor and seek professional help.

16 Depression Induction

The following may be adapted for people who prefer a more active approach. Normally I count upwards when inducing trance and in the reverse order when exiting however in this instance it seems more applicable to start by counting down. You, the reader may use whichever method suits best.

Sit down and settle back nice and comfortably, then take a slow deep breath and close your eyes. Imagine with your eyes closed that you are focusing on the tip of your nose, concentrating on the tip of your nose and as you do so breathe slowly and deeply 5 times, making sure to hold the air for several seconds before exhaling. On each exhalation tell yourself that you're going deeper and deeper into hypnosis.

Leave a long enough pause for the breathing.

Now relax your eyes and imagine you are on the top (5th) floor in a very lavish, hotel elevator which is going down to ground level and as it passes through each level you go deeper and deeper into trance. 5- level 5, the floor of the elevator has plush carpeting and you feel your feet sinking into the soft material as the elevator moves down and down. 4 - 4th level, letting go still more. The pattern and color of the carpet fascinates you and there is the sound of soft music, which you find pleasing to the ear and this helps to relax you even more. 3-3rd level, deeper, deeper relaxed. There is a pleasant fragrance, which is light and vaguely familiar and you find the smooth, downward motion of the elevator strangely comforting. 2-2nd level, almost at your destination deeply relaxed and 1-level 1, the elevator door opens and the hotel foyer leads out to your favorite place. It could be on the top of a mountain ready to ski, at a swimming pool or ocean ready to swim, inside a gym ready to work out. Perhaps it's sitting by the fire in a cozy cottage relaxing and watching TV, listening to the radio, painting or playing the piano. Perhaps it's in a forest preparing to jog, cycle or hike. Spend two minutes of clock time imagining the activity and as you do so you slip deeper and deeper into comfort and trance.

If you would rather have a scripted activity you may use the following if applicable.

It is a warm spring day, the sun is high in the sky and it sparkles and dances on the soft snow beneath. It seems as if the white powder has tiny diamonds in it reflecting and refracting the light. You lift up a handful of snow and marvel at its soft powdery texture. The cool mountain air feels like peppermint on your cheeks and the world seems silent, no sounds, no people here, for this is your special place. Standing at the peak you survey all around you, the snow covered evergreens, the ocean far off in the distance and the city with its seemingly miniature buildings miles and miles away. It looks as if the ski run stretches endlessly, the air smells crisp and fresh and the conditions for skiing are ideal. You adjust your ski mask and brace yourself for what lies ahead, then you push off with your poles and down you go. Gliding and swishing, swishing and gliding, the fresh mountain air and the speed are intoxicatingly delightful.

Take a 2-minute pause to enjoy your favorite activity and this deepens the trance.

Joy comes from many sources: places, people, activities and pets and sometimes animals seem to understand us more than we understand ourselves. When we are sick it is easy to feel sorry for ourselves and to think negatively but in order to regain mental and physical harmony it is important to stop our negative thinking and conjure up pleasant thoughts instead.

If you have a pet now or one from the past, a dog or a cat that you loved very much, imagine stroking your pet, enjoying the texture of its coat, the warmth of its body by your side, the affection it gives/gave so freely, loving you totally, totally loving. It's complete and utter acceptance, soothing and reassuring. And the sound of my voice and each and every exhalation continues to take you deeper and deeper into comfort and trance.

Now imagine creating a scrapbook with your pet snuggling up beside you, a scrapbook of the future the way you would like it to be once you are well again. Imagine yourself spending time with the people you love and enjoy. Become aware of the activities you are choosing to participate in… View the places you are going to…

See yourself, strong and robust once more, full of vitality, completely recovered. Fill in all the details of these future images, the sights, smells, tastes, textures and sounds and feel the joy.

You are looking forward manifesting the life you desire, inspired by what lies ahead and it feels good.

You are recovering, getting stronger and stronger every day. Your mind is extremely powerful, you use it to your advantage, you want to get well quickly and you will get well quickly. Focus on positive thoughts and see yourself in the future happy, healthy, and vibrant.

Now enjoy your special place for a few moments longer then I am going to count from 1 up to 5 and when I reach the number 5 you will come back to full conscious awareness feeling very, very good. **One**, *you have done some good work today and you are learning how to use the power of your subconscious mind to help and heal yourself.* **Two**, *each and every time you choose to do this kind of therapy, whether with me or another hypnotherapist or listening to your recording you will go deeper and faster than the time before.* **Three**, *you will gain great healing benefits and enjoy the process immensely.* **Four**, *slowly, gently, normal sensation returning to your body and you may wiggle your fingers and your toes and* **Five**, *returning to full conscious awareness, aware again of the sounds in the room and eyes open, wide, wide awake feeling absolutely marvelous. If you like, give yourself a positive mental suggestion as you reorient back to the room.*

17 Switching Off

You may use any of the italicized introductory inductions to preface the suggestions in this script.

Continue to take a nice deep breath and relax, and now that your body is relaxed your mind needs to slow down and relax too. Imagine all your cares and concerns flowing away from you like rays of light radiating outwards. And as they move outwards you feel a sense of relief and release, while the sound of my voice and each and every exhalation takes you deeper and deeper into comfort and trance. Imagine that it's time to take a vacation, a long overdue vacation, and this can be your ideal vacation. Perhaps it's to a real place that you have already visited or maybe it's somewhere you hope to visit in the future. Maybe a tropical island, snow covered mountains, a forested region or a countryside location with green meadows and undulating hills. Take a few moments to decide where you will go… see the place, the colors, the details… smell the fragrances, the aromas, the scents… feel the sensation of being in this place and enjoy these pleasurable feelings… I will be quiet for one minute of clock time to allow you to enjoy this place and as you do so you will slip deeper and deeper into comfort and trance.

Pause for one minute.

Now imagine a veritable feast set out before you, there's every type of food imaginable. Bowls of fruit of different varieties and colors, soups, savory dishes, roasts of meat, fish, pastas, curries, steaks, fresh crisp salads, roasted vegetables, cold cuts and deserts. Decorative and enticing, something for every taste. Perhaps your appetizer will be a warm soothing soup, or a crispy fresh salad… and your entrée a flavorful medley of delight. Your desert a sweet treat, creamy and light… or a plate of fresh fruit…bite into it and notice the texture. Is it soft, crispy, crunchy, does it taste salty, sweet, bitter, sour, or tangy? In a moment I will be quiet for one minute of clock time to allow you to choose and enjoy this sumptuous feast and as you do so you will slip deeper and deeper into comfort and trance.

Pause for one minute.

Now you are fully satisfied and you choose to rest for a while in order to digest your food. Perhaps you lie on the beach listening to the rhythmic sound of the waves lulling you to sleep and feeling the gentle warmth of the sun caressing your body… Maybe you settle down in the warmth of a cozy cottage high up in the snowy mountains as you survey the pristine white landscape outside. You're just drifting and drowsy, drowsy and drifting, floating deeper and deeper into comfort and trance. So wonderful to feel this physical and mental comfort, nothing to do, no one to please just let yourself be.

Later you choose to participate in your favorite activity walking, swimming, skiing, reading, sailing, whatever appeals to you. And it's wonderful to spend time enjoying this activity.

Pause for 1 minute.

And finally it's evening and again you choose how you wish to spend your time, with or without company. Do you want to be entertained… laugh with or at comedians? Watch dancers or acrobats perform? Marvel at the beauty and skill of their physical abilities or would you rather become enthralled with soft or rousing music? Perhaps you want to sit quietly under the stars or watch a movie. The choice is yours and while you relax and enjoy your evening for a few minutes the pleasure of this perfect vacation intensifies and stays with you long after you awaken from this induction.

Allow 2 minutes of silence.

Now enjoy your special place for a few moments longer then I am going to count from 5 down to 1 and when I reach the number 1 you will come back to full conscious awareness feeling very, very good. **Five***, you have done some good work today and you are learning how to use the power of your subconscious mind to help and heal yourself.* **Four,** *each and every time you choose to do this kind of therapy, whether with me or another hypnotherapist or listening to your recording you will go deeper and faster than the time before.* **Three,** *you will gain great healing benefits and enjoy the process immensely.* **Two,** *slowly, gently, normal sensation returning to your body and you may wiggle your fingers and your toes and* **One,** *returning to full conscious awareness, aware again of the sounds in the room and eyes open, wide, wide awake feeling absolutely marvelous. If you like you can give yourself a positive mental suggestion as you reorient back to the room.*

18 The Old Curiosity Shop-Gaining Insight

Use any of the italicized introductory inductions to preface the suggestions in this script.

And now that you are so comfortably relaxed you sit down by a grassy bank and survey the landscape in front of you. There is a long winding path and you decide to follow it walking at a slow, steady pace until you find yourself standing outside an old building with a sign that reads, 'Ye Old Curiosity Shop — selling antique and modern artifacts.' Intrigued you peer inside the glass and see a variety of interesting items, globes, scales, paintings and ornaments. Wanting to see more you are drawn inside the softly lit interior. And every thought, every sound, every sensation takes you deeper still.

You stand in the centre of the room enjoying the ambience, aware of the fragrant scent of incense and the soft sound of what seems to be wind chimes. There are curiosities from all around the world, exotic tapestries, beautiful crystals, and ornate statues. The owner of the store, an old man with silver hair and grey overalls greets you warmly and encourages you to browse. You do so for several minutes enjoying the various treasures.

Allow 2 minutes of silence to deepen the trance.

After a while the old man points to a shelf with lucky charms, horseshoes, leprechauns, guardian angels and dream catchers and he asks you to examine each charm in detail. Pick up the first lucky charm, the horseshoe, notice the color of the metal, how many nail holes it has, does it shine and sparkle or is it old and rusty?... How big is it, is it heavy or light?... The old man tells you that horseshoes are believed to be protective. This is because they are crescent shaped, which, according to legend represent a variety of moon goddesses who were protective. He asks you to consider what kind of protection you need and you spend some time pondering the thought.

Allow one minute of silence.

Now pick up the second lucky charm, the leprechaun, what does this fairy cobbler look like, is his beard long or short, his clothes green or red? ... Do his shoes have buckles? ... Is he heavy or light? ... What is he made of? ... The store-owner tells you that people believe if you hold onto a leprechaun he will give you three wishes, so long as you promise to release him. The old man asks you what you wish for apart from the obvious ... He tells you to look deeper.

Allow one minute of silence.

You move on to examine the guardian angel noting what he/she looks like, the material the charm is made of, its color and whether or not it is heavy or light. The owner of the store says that throughout antiquity people have believed that guardian angels protect and guide and he asks you what kind of guidance you need.

Allow one minute of silence.

Finally your gaze falls upon the dream catcher and you lift it up and examine the hoop, the weave and the feathers. What colors are the feathers are they large or small? The old man says that Native Americans believe the dream catcher protects us while we sleep, stopping bad dreams and only allowing good dreams to pass through. Imagine, for a moment, that all your fears are stopped by the dream catcher – and only your hopes and wishes materialize. What will you do differently in your future life when your health is restored?

Allow one minute of silence.

The old man hands you a bracelet with miniature charms of the items you have been looking at, he smiles warmly and says it is his gift to you and will bring you luck. You are touched by his kindness and are thanking him profusely when a cool breeze brushes against your cheek. Slowly opening your eyes, you realize you have been asleep and the encounter was all a dream. The winding path still lies in front of you but somehow you know that the next part of your journey will be much easier.

Now enjoy your special place for a few moments longer then I am going to count from 5 down to 1 and when I reach the number 1 you will come back to full conscious awareness feeling very, very good. ***Five****, you have done some good work today and you are learning how to use the* *power of your subconscious mind to help and heal yourself.* **Four,** *each and every time you choose to do this kind of therapy, whether with me or another hypnotherapist or listening to your recording you will go deeper and faster than the time before.* **Three,** *you will gain great healing benefits and enjoy the process immensely.* **Two,** *slowly, gently, normal sensation returning to your body and you may wiggle your fingers and your toes and* **One,** *returning to full conscious awareness, aware again of the sounds in the room and eyes open wide, wide awake feeling absolutely marvelous. If you like you can give yourself a positive mental suggestion as you reorient back to the room.*

19 Reflections-Inner Resources

You may use any of the italicized introductory inductions to preface the suggestions in this script.

Imagine stepping into a room with three large mirrors, each mirror is rectangular in shape and at least six feet high. Look at the centre mirror and see that it has a sign above it which reads, 'The Present,' now look over to the mirror on the left and notice the sign above it, which says, 'The Past,' and finally look at the mirror on the right which reads, 'The Future.'

And every thought, every sound, every sensation takes you deeper and deeper into comfort and trance.

On the floor in the middle of the room is a large brass plaque with instructions engraved in gold letters. Look closely at the words and read them aloud. *'Whosoever stands on this plaque will be made aware of their own inner strengths in the present. That person may review how these have been used in the past and how they may prove helpful in the future, by simply looking into the appropriate mirror.'*

And every thought, every sound, every sensation takes you deeper and deeper into comfort and trance.

Intrigued you stand on the plaque in front of the centre mirror and to your amazement glowing letters begin to appear on the surface. These eventually come together and form a word or words, which denote one of your strengths. Perhaps it's intelligence... kindness... creativity ... athleticism ... patience ... sociability ... or any other quality, it really doesn't matter which strength it is so long as it's relevant for you.

And every thought, every sound, every sensation takes you deeper and deeper into comfort and trance.

Now turn towards the mirror on the left, the mirror that represents the past and stare at your reflection. Slowly the mirror's surface comes to life, colors begin to swirl around and eventually they form moving pictures of how you utilized this strength to help you in the past.

Mesmerized you watch as memories of past successes slowly come into your awareness and delight you.

Pause for one minute.

And every thought, every sound, every sensation takes you deeper and deeper into comfort and trance.

When the movie ends you are ready to face the mirror on your right, the mirror which represents the future and to stare at your reflection. Slowly, almost imperceptibly at first the colors swirl around and eventually future possibilities unfold, ways of dealing with challenges, ways that you hadn't considered before. Enjoy watching these future movies for as long as you need and know that any time you need to overcome apparently insurmountable challenges you may visit the mirror room and gain great insight into your own resources.

Pause for two minutes.

Now enjoy your special place for a few moments longer then I am going to count from 5 down to 1 and when I reach the number 1 you will come back to full conscious awareness feeling very, very good. **Five**, *you have done some good work today and you are learning how to use the power of your subconscious mind to help and heal yourself.* **Four,** *each and every time you choose to do this kind of therapy, whether with me or another hypnotherapist or listening to your recording you will go deeper and faster than the time before.* **Three,** *you will gain great healing benefits and enjoy the process immensely.* **Two,** *slowly, gently, normal sensation returning to your body and you may wiggle your fingers and your toes and* **One,** *returning to full conscious awareness, aware again of the sounds in the room and eyes open, wide, wide awake, feeling absolutely marvelous. If you like you can give yourself a positive mental suggestion as you reorient back to the room.*

20 Self Hypnosis Induction

This should never be used in conjunction with any other activity like driving or operating machinery. Your entire attention should only be on the induction.

Depending on how you are feeling and how active you are during treatment there may be times when you are not in the comfort of your own home but still want to reinforce your hypnosis. If this is the case then you will find it helpful to practice self-hypnosis for a few minutes two or three times a day. Find a quiet location if possible and if not just find somewhere that you can sit down and be undisturbed for a short time. Next, locate a spot for your eyes to focus on, it can be a mark on the wall, a doorknob, a flower, anything at all that you can simply stare at. Take a few slow, deep breaths and then begin to imagine relaxation flowing through your body from the top of your head to the tips of your toes. Some people imagine a beautiful color passing through their bodies and as that color touches different parts of the body the muscles relax. Others imagine tensing and relaxing different pairs of muscles groups, for example, the biceps and the triceps, or you can imagine a warm liquid travelling from the top of your head to the tips of your toes. Some simply tell themselves that their body is warm and relaxed – whichever method suits you, the idea is to help yourself to physically relax.

The second part is to deepen the experience by imagining a staircase with 10 steps going downwards and as you step down each step imagine yourself going deeper into hypnosis. You may also tell yourself that even the count itself will take you deeper still. Some people prefer to think of themselves floating upwards towards the stars and as they float they slip deeper and deeper into hypnosis. Again it will be a matter of preference as to your choice and of course you can create your own scenarios.

The final touch (before adding your positive suggestions or affirmations) is to imagine a beautiful or favorite place where you can spend some time and to utilize all of your senses to make the experience more vivid. If for instance you choose a lovely beach then you can ask yourself what would I see in this place, what would I hear, smell, taste and touch? The more detailed the imagery the more relaxed you will feel.

Once you have gone through these procedures you can give yourself positive suggestions such as. "My body is healing and I am getting stronger and stronger every day. My powerful immune system is destroying any cancer cells. I release all fears and anxieties. I am able to eat and sleep well." Create your own suggestions and whenever possible use positive language so rather than say, "I don't feel sick anymore," say, "I feel healthy now." Whenever possible keep your suggestions in the present tense and see yourself cancer free doing all the things you love to do. The entire process takes only a few minutes and enhances the work you are doing at home. Don't worry if it's noisy where you are as you can incorporate any sounds around you into your induction by telling yourself that all external sounds take you deeper and deeper into hypnosis.

Finally bring yourself out of hypnosis by using the counting out induction.

11: Interlives

Why is cancer so frightening?

I believe that part of the reason may be our fear of impending death, particularly for people who are non religious, but what if we really don't die, what if we reincarnate many times?

In order to help overcome my own fear of death (even though I believe in God) I decided to explore past lives using hypnotherapy. In addition I examined clients' interlives that is the time between one life and the next. In essence, I looked at what happens to the soul while it is in the spiritual dimension.

If reincarnation and life between lives exist then my fear of death would be diminished. I therefore dedicate this chapter of the book to accounts given by clients who under hypnosis recall the interlives they experienced. Perhaps their descriptions will help allay some of your fears.

Twenty years ago a woman, Rona, entered my office and told me she had been suffering from a phobia all of her life.

Rona asked me for help and wanted to try hypnosis to cure the problem so after some discussion I put Rona into a trance and asked her subconscious mind to take her to the origin of the problem. Imagine my surprise when she regressed into a past life and re-experienced the trauma which she believed had caused her phobia. After the session Rona left my office convinced that her phobia was gone and to this day she remains phobia-free.

That was my introduction to past life regression. It had not been my intention to take the client into a past life, instead I was expecting her to regress to an incident in this lifetime, but even so it made me aware of the power of this type of therapy. Since then, I have regressed many people and found that it helped them gain insight and sometimes resolution for a variety of issues. Individual past lives are diverse, ranging from exciting to humdrum, happy to sad and traumatic to non eventful.

As my expertise grew, I also hypnotized people to visit that period of time between one incarnation and the next, which is generally referred to as the interlife.

In essence, I explored what might happen when people die, where they go and what transpires before they reincarnate. As a cancer survivor I find these stories encouraging and want to share some of them with you the reader.

I summarize these narratives and occasionally improve them grammatically to increase comprehension but I do not change the content. Of course we cannot know the validity of the accounts, is it just the brain playing a trick on us or is it real, that is up to the individual to ascertain but I believe it may give some of us hope and ultimately peace of mind.

Before delving into the interlife, I'll include one past life in this chapter because it's relevant to our topic at hand. Past lives however are usually so specific that it's difficult to draw common themes that are helpful to the general public.

I'll begin by looking at what Deborah, a member of my cancer group, found on exploring a past life during trance:

"I am a teacher on the board of health and studying cancer, researching. I see myself wearing white moccasins, a long dress, and wire rimmed glasses. I am

Caucasian about 35 years of age and I am in a huge library doing research. Looking outside the window I see people walking and riding bicycles, along a dirt road in a village. A newspaper in the library says it is March 18th, 1864. I think I'm in England. My mother is a doctor, my father a builder and I'm married with 3 children, aged five, seven and eight, two daughters and a son. We all live in the same house, and my husband is a writer. He writes mystery novels. My name is Catherine Black and I have found that there is a cure for cancer using our own plants, in fact I have written a book about it. I knew that plants could help to heal so I spent a great deal of time doing research on plants like Cat's Claw, Horseradish and Burdock..."

Now, therapy sessions do not last forever and due to time constraints, I often have to move clients on through their lives and ask them to identify any major events. This was the case with Deborah and I asked her to scan through the years and summarise her findings. She did so but unfortunately near the end of her life Deborah became extremely distraught because the villagers burned her book, the only copy she had, as they believed it to be witchcraft.

I calmed Deborah down and moved her through that lifetime so she was able to enter into the interlife, that is the period of time between her past life and the next life. Here is her account:

"I am floating it's very peaceful, it's bright and everything is white but there are no colours. Other bodies are floating too, there are no faces which is kind of odd. I think we are in a holding place, it's tranquil and I see more and more of us now. Around and outside are white buildings and we are learning something, healing ourselves and meditating."

Clients in the interlife enjoy spending considerable time in one place but wanting to know more I move Deborah forward and ask what she is aware of. *"Now I am in a peaceful garden full of wonderful colours and I feel very calm as I walk through the garden... there is no sense of time and I see a beautiful waterfall."*

Deborah wanted to stay in this garden while in trance but I again moved her forward to find out what happened next.

"Now I am just learning and everyone is so loving. We are allowed to choose our next life and I choose to be a healer but I have to wait."

At this point our time was up and I had to bring Deborah out of trance but it's interesting to note that in this lifetime she's actually experienced the disease she was researching.

In the narratives that follow you will find similarities as well as differences.

Gabriel is a professional man in his forties and he gives a descriptive account of his experience of the afterlife:

"There are two aspects, the first is when I am awakened from the experience of death, the background is black and I'm surrounded by luminous bubbles some are white and some pastel in color. I'm not standing on anything probably because I don't have feet. I'm in spirit form ... I am amongst different bubbles like soap bubbles but these are soft, they are tangible and they can bend around. They remind me of the big feathery things that showgirls wear. It's not as if there is light shining on me, the whole place is bright, I feel like I am surrounded by these bubbles of light, they are all over me, they are all around me. They don't feel like they are physical, not as if you are walking through soft grass or big feathers yet they feel more substantial than light.

The second aspect when we were doing the regression, when I was in spirit form, I had visions of being pulled by my neck, my back lapel and just flying around. If I had wanted to go somewhere else I couldn't because some force was pulling me over and above the bubbles. I was flying across the bubbles, not in a linear sense and I had access to all the bubbles at the same time if I wanted. It wasn't like a narrow path. During these experiences I was going through the impressions of what I know. These bubbles represented my past lives, they kind of formed a time line. It was as if I was flying in the sky and I saw a traffic jam on the highway. In that flight I also saw what I was familiar with and when I was reviewing my incarnations I still had vestiges of memory."

Gabriel felt extremely peaceful and content during his experience, as did the next subject, Kelly.

Kelly is a young, professional woman in her twenties. During trance it was difficult for Kelly to relay what was happening so upon reawakening she gave the following account:

"I feel like everything was happening so fast, it's difficult to describe it. I could talk, I could have conversations, I could see it vividly, it is a strange experience. I saw these flashes and it looked like a screen that faded into black. It seemed like a monitor of some kind. I saw the room, then it just faded away and I saw balls of bluish, navy bluish light, they were moving so quickly and I didn't know how much time had passed. I could feel the balls of light and I could hear some voices, kind of faint but I wasn't scared and someone was talking to me.

All of a sudden, the ground disappeared and there were people, so many people, kids and older people, I could see them vividly and they had bodies and clothing on. I could talk to them and asked, "Who are you? What are you doing?" and "Why am I here?" and they said they were waiting for me. "What do you mean?" I asked and they said, "Well you're here now, it's over you're here with us." "Where is this?" I asked and sometimes it was a man who would respond to me and at other times it was a woman. I heard a ladies voice say, "You're here now and we're here to take you through it." I didn't understand what was going on... then it just faded away and it was darker but I wasn't scared I felt at peace.

And then there was light, I couldn't tell where it was and there was a ground of some sort. I could feel people, other souls and I could feel energy but I didn't have a physical body. I couldn't look down, I couldn't see anything and felt I couldn't really control where I was going. There were flashes of the physical world that I was going through, I could see somebody, then a mountain range and then again another flash. I didn't feel like I had any emotions, no emotions, nothing, but I always had this white light behind my eyes. When I noticed people, they didn't look like people, they seemed to be glowing. It wasn't like I was seeing somebody in real life. It was as if I was watching someone on TV, but they were glowing and they were all smiling and happy."

It seems that Kelly was very much aware of what happened immediately after death and in the early stages of her interlife.

However, Ivy, a member of my cancer group might be relaying what happens a little later on in the journey. Here is Ivy's account:

"We are outside, it looks like a school, or a university. There are other people, I know them but I don't know what we're doing, we're just outside a place of learning. (Ivy is spending a long time enjoying her visit but I'm aware of time constraints in session so I count from 1-3 to move her forward and ask what happens next).

We're in a classroom now, it's like a lecture but I don't know what it's about. (She chuckles and I ask why) Girls on one side, boys on the other. People look the same as people on earth and I feel so happy. (Again I count from 1-3 to move Ivy forward and accelerate the process) Ah, it's like a cloud, like not being on the ground, it's sunny, there are other people and they are familiar, they are nice and happy.

I don't know what we are doing, we are just there and everything is white and gold. (She falls silent for a while so I move her forward again). It's not as bright anymore and I'm by myself but not lonely.

I don't have a physical body and I feel like I'm floating but I don't have to go anywhere because I can see a long way into the distance. There is no real time and I don't talk but I know when conversation happens. I am just watching, not doing anything and I can see the beginning of life like sunrise.

I'm by myself feeling good, just being. There's nothing to feel bad about. Before I reincarnate I'm aware of golden light coming over the horizon."

The one theme that keeps repeating is the peacefulness every one of these subjects feels. In two of the following accounts subjects meet loved ones on the other side.

Pearl, now in her seventies is a retired therapist and this is what she experienced:

"I saw David (her current partner in this lifetime) in the hallway and he was smiling and we walked down the corridor together, hand in hand. Then he said he had to go but he would come back. I wandered outside and saw my girlfriend who was in a flower garden, so I joined her and we spent time together enjoying the flowers. She was sprinkling them with water. The water is different to what we have here, it formed a beautiful sparkly mist and I watched it for a while. Afterwards we went out towards the gate and there were people, lots of people and somebody rode by on a bicycle. I couldn't really see the ground but the people were all able to walk on something. I walked to the gate, and then David showed up and he was smiling and we were happy to see each other again."

Kayla is 26-years-old and is studying psychology and wants to work in the criminal justice system.

Kayla is eager to explore what exists in the interlife so I put her into a deep trance and ask, "What are your first impressions?" She responds: *"There are some colors, greens, it's very calm, people don't seem to notice me, daily lives are calm. There's no stress, no time, lack of time is nice. Everyone is on their own path, they are moving at their own pace, deciding where to go, together or separately. I feel it's different from what I expect heaven to be like when I die, because it seems lower to the earth. The background is black and there are bubbles, I think they are possible future lifetimes and you have to jump into one of them. I wonder if we get to choose where we go?*

Unfortunately time constraints exist so it is not always possible for me to meet with subjects and glean more information but by accumulating different narratives you the reader can get a glimpse into the unknown. Judy's account of the afterlife is brief yet beautifully descriptive:

"There's yellow, gold and purple light and there are people all around, there are so many of them they look like dust almost like sand. The environment is made of beautiful crystals and I see angels floating in the air and hear soothing, relaxing music. Dad is here to meet me and there's a beautiful lady with porcelain skin and blue eyes. She is holding a book, I don't know what it is about but I know I have to learn something from that book and it has to do with making a choice."

My last account of these narratives comes from Robin a woman in her sixties who is both an intuitive healer in this lifetime and a channeler. Robin agreed to explore her interlife while under hypnosis. During trance she found it difficult to speak and when she did so her voice was labored and almost inaudible.

Upon her wakening I asked Robin to relay her experience. The following is her account:

"The energy was everywhere all around, circular, lots of color, there was no body form of any sort, it was like consciousness as opposed to having to take any form. I could feel when I hugged somebody but it's not like physically hugging somebody it's the way the energy would

change, there would be circular colors and movement in waves.

In the hug with another energy form I felt that the energy seemed to move in horizontal waves and the movement was constant. I felt the vibrations and I saw the waves. It helps me to understand a part of my personality, the part that really tries to live in the moment because being there was just being there.

It wasn't about being an artist or getting creativity out in a certain way, it just was. Every second of life was creativity and it's not like creating a thought or a form, it's just being. It's all about being and being in the moment and I think that's the way I am because I don't plan ahead.

There was no angst, anxiety, or stress it was just so comfortable and it takes away the pressure this life puts on people. No attachment, not lonely though, that was the furthest thing from what I felt. I felt so close to everything, all the energy around me.

There was a different physicality when I was happy to see someone. There was a blending. I remember my passing and I thought wow we time this and this is supposed to be.

I also remember the thought of connecting, going over a lifetime and it was so brief because it was unnecessary since being discarnate is a different type of consciousness .

If I were to draw it, it would be circular and there would be no separation between energies. It's not like somebody had to go gardening or perform a task, I never saw a separateness to any other energy.

Colors are very vibrant impossible to paint because there are no colors here to that degree of vibrancy and aliveness.

This place of spirit is all energy and feeling. I was so present and so happy. To me I was constantly active so full and beautiful. I felt like I was speaking in another tongue though I know I was speaking in English but it felt like I was from somewhere else.

I remember looking into a future lifetime and being very resistant. All of a sudden I was being guided and they said they really needed me to go. It felt as if there was no time, I could have been there for ten years, it was timeless and I didn't want to leave and take another lifetime, I was so happy to be back there, it felt so right. Nevertheless it has given me a greater understanding of my DNA.

I was given a choice to reincarnate between two bodies and I chose this current body I am in because she is such a gentle person, her energy is light and she is extremely sensitive. Coming from that other place makes me understand why when I really love something I'm intensely passionate and creative."

The above accounts are fascinating and exploring the interlife helped my clients in different ways. For some it eliminated the fear of death and for others it allowed them to gain a greater understanding of themselves.

Now it is definitely not my intention to paint a picture of this wonderful interlife experience and encourage people to think that death is preferable to being ill and therefore end their lives. That is the furthest thing from my mind and it would be senseless because the truth is no one really knows what's on the other side.

My intention, through my findings, is merely to give hope to those who are afraid of death and to those who are terminally ill with cancer. Just as hope springs eternal perhaps life does too.

12: Conclusion

Throughout this book my predominant focus has been on cancer patients and cancer survivors.

We do not however live in isolation and our struggle has a ripple effect, which spreads outwards affecting our families, friends and society in general.

Family members, partners and children are often terrified when they hear that their loved one has cancer. Some, despite their own misgivings are protective and manage to act in a calm, contained manner assuring the patient that all will be well, while others openly show their dismay.

Certain friends and neighbors are able to rally round supportively but some don't know how to respond, they are uncomfortable and fear saying the wrong thing so they avoid contact.

Partners and caregivers have to take on more responsibility, doing additional chores, and accompanying their loved ones to endless medical appointments and this puts tremendous stress on everyone. It's important therefore that family members other than just the identified patient reach out to free support groups and additional resources.

When I was sick my oldest daughter told her coworkers about the situation at home and she was amazed, as was I, at the kindness these people displayed, people who had never even met me. Some shared inspirational stories about cancer survivors, others, who had themselves survived cancer, offered to phone me with words of encouragement.

Still others sent recipes for juicing and preparing healthy meals. These offerings really helped particularly the phone calls from people who had beaten cancer and appeared to be enjoying life again. If you don't know any cancer survivors you can find a telephone mentor online, a volunteer who has gone through cancer and has been trained to help support you. Being able to voice your concerns to someone who really understands is a godsend.

When I started my small hypnotherapy group for cancer patients and survivors I thought the members would benefit from hypnosis and of course they did however much to my surprise I also benefitted. Talking and sharing with people who had been through the same experience as I had was both healing and informative. A camaraderie of sorts developed between all of us and I genuinely look forward to our weekly meetings.

Interestingly, over the years, past clients have told me that while undergoing cancer treatment they felt nurtured, looked after and cared for.

Despite the negative aspects of the experience they received a lot of positive attention from medical staff, family and friends and when the all clear was given and they were cancer free the attention stopped. Everyone just expected them to get on with their lives as before, resume where they left off but on every level mentally, physically, emotionally and spiritually they had changed and still needed help to transition. A void had been created so I worked with these people to seek the supports they needed and encouraged them to utilize complementary therapies they believed would be beneficial.

Before cancer I was working part-time as a school counselor and could not use my hypnotherapy skills in that setting. But with the onset of the disease I chose to retire from the school district. This freed me up to spend more time working with hypnotherapy, a modality that I have always felt passionate about. Most clients wanted help with anxiety, depression and habit disorders like overeating and smoking, but some wanted to explore their past lives and interlives. I found this work fascinating and it is wonderful in the sense that it gives some people hope that life after death is a possibility, thus diminishing the fear of death.

Our belief system impacts our mood and our health and when I was at my weakest, hypnotherapy really helped me to feel safe, comfortable and hopeful. That is why I have included several chapters of hypnotherapy scripts in the text.

I like to imagine that inside each of us is a tiny spark, a spark that can be ignited, by prayer, meditation, hypnotherapy, or communing with nature.

Imagine that spark turning into a brilliant light, a light that connects us to a power greater than self, God, the divine, universal energy, whatever you want to call it, a healing, benevolent light. Hypnotherapy harnesses our imagination and allows us to use the power of the subconscious mind for healing.

Now my way of coping with cancer is obviously not the only way to go and the members of my cancer group were good enough to share their stories with me in the hope that their experiences will help others.

Remember Deborah? Despite the shock of receiving a cancer diagnosis Deborah had the strength to disagree with her first oncologist, who had advised her to have a mastectomy. She instead found a different doctor whose beliefs matched her own. This doctor performed a lumpectomy and Deborah felt good about the surgery.

Afterwards, Deborah decided against chemotherapy and radiation. Instead she changed her diet completely consulting a herbalist/nutritionist and becoming vegan. In addition Deborah received oxygen therapy, did exercises and meditated and is now cancer free.

Ivy followed the conventional course of treatment initially but when the cancer returned years later she began taking experimental drugs and is still doing so. Ivy keeps herself busy and distracted and says her faith in God and the support of family are the most important things in her life. Linda also followed traditional treatment when she was first diagnosed with cancer but when it returned years later she combined complementary therapies like Hyperthermia and was pleased with the results.

Alex had chemotherapy for Non Hodgkin lymphoma and received a stem cell transplant. Although currently cancer-free he is still undergoing chemotherapy and says cancer has strengthened his faith in God. He also feels greatly supported by his family. Of course it's good to hear from people who have been cancer-free for a long period of time and to listen to the reasons they give for having had a long and healthy life. Judy is one such person, following conventional treatment she took Tamoxifen for five years, and has been cancer-free for 26 years. She believes that being busy and optimistic is the key to success.

Before drawing this book to a close, I would like to thank the B.C. Cancer Agency for the treatment I received, it helped save my life and I will be forever grateful. The oncologists and medical staff were fantastic, and I believe in traditional treatment because it is research based. Their website offers a wealth of information.

My own oncologist in Richmond is also one of the kindest men I have ever met. He is compassionate and extremely knowledgeable. He has helped me tremendously.

For many people conventional treatments are not the way they want to go and they choose a drug free, more natural approach. If there's one thing that being a therapist has taught me it is that we are all different and there are many ways to deal with any one problem.

Whichever path you choose, it is advisable to be proactive, become informed, find out what options you have and educate yourself. I hope some of the tools in this book will empower you to travel through your own unique journey with courage and determination. Remember you're not alone, so reach out and embrace all your supports.

As I've said previously, use the things that help you and discard the rest. Having said that however I strongly believe complementary treatments should be used in addition to mainstream medicine in order to enhance recovery.

I recommend hypnotherapy in *addition* to conventional treatment, not as a substitute. Hypnotherapy helps with pain management and healing. It can address anxiety and depression and is something we can do when the rest of our body is at its weakest. Moreover, it is non-invasive.

As I finish this book I see the faces of the people I know who have or have had cancer, some are young and some are old, but we are all hopeful. We represent mankind and we want to live.

For me, the cancer conundrum was a wakeup call, one that forced me to make difficult choices around treatment and life's priorities. It taught me to slow down and appreciate the good things I have… They say every cloud has a silver lining – what's yours?

About the Author

Louise Evans B.A., M.Ed., C.Ht., R.C.C., has worked for the past 20 years as a hypnotherapist/counselor in private practice. (www.sparkhypnotherapy.com / www.louiserevans.com)

She has two office locations in British Columbia, one in Kitsilano and one in Metrotown.

Louise has dual citizenship as a Canadian Citizen and a British Subject and has lived in Canada since 1979.

Originally from Scotland she graduated with a BA degree and a Teaching Certificate and upon immigrating to Canada taught sciences at the secondary level for several years.

After marriage Louise stopped working for a while in order to take care of her four children and during that time she became interested in hypnotherapy and counseling. As a result, Louise trained with the Canadian Society of Clinical Hypnosis (BC Division). She obtained her Masters in Counseling Psychology at UBC and became a Master Clinical Hypnotherapist at the Pacific Institute of Advanced Hypnotherapy. The latter is the only school in Canada, which offers a hypnosis-training course in the family medicine program at Alberta University, which is accredited as a recognized elective.

Since then she has trained with some of the best teachers in the world including Roy Hunter, Cal Banyon, Dr. Brian Weiss, Dr. Bruce Eimer, Dr. Yapko and Dr. Karen Olness. Louise continues to attend workshops and lectures.

Hypnotherapy also helps her on a personal level to be comfortable presenting in front of large audiences and in surviving cancer. Louise Evans has been cancer-free since 2015 and lives with her husband in Vancouver. You may contact Louise at: Lshanter@shaw.ca

References

Hypnosis on anxiety in patients with cancer: A Chen, P., Liu, Y., & Chen, M. (2017). The effect of Meta-Analysis. *Worldviews on Evidence-Based Nursing, 14*(3) 223-236 doi:10.1111/wvn.12215

Elkins, G., Johnson, A., & Fisher, W. (2012). Cognitive hypnotherapy for pain management.*American Journal of Clinical Hypnosis, 54*(4), 294-310 doi:10.1080/00029157.….654284

Maclaughlan David, S., Salzillo, S., Bowe, P., Scuncio, S., Malit, B., Raker, C., . . . Dizon, D. S. (2013). Randomised controlled trial comparing hypnotherapy versus gabapentin for the treatment of hot flashes in breast cancer survivors: A pilot study. *BMJ Open, 3*(9), e003138. doi:10.1136/bmjopen-2013-003138

Sharma, V. (2017). Hypnotherapy in cancer care: Clinical benefits and prospective implications. *Journal of Health Research & Reviews, 4*(3) doi:10.4103/jhrr.jhrr_45_17

Téllez A, Juárez-García D M, Jaime-Bernal L, Medina De la Garza C E, Sánchez T. (2017). The effect of hypnotherapy on the quality of life in women with breast cancer. *Psychology in Russia, 10*(2), 144-240. doi:10.11621/pir.2017.0216

Téllez, A., Rodríguez-Padilla, C., Martínez-Rodríguez, J. L., Juárez-García, D. M., Sanchez-Armass, O., Sánchez, T., Jaime-Bernal, L. (2017). Psychological effects of group hypnotherapy on breast cancer patients during chemotherapy. *American Journal of Clinical Hypnosis, 60*(1), 68. doi:10.1080/00029157.2016.1210497

BC Cancer Agency: www.bccancer.bc.ca

Manor House
905-648-2193
www.manor-house-publishing.com

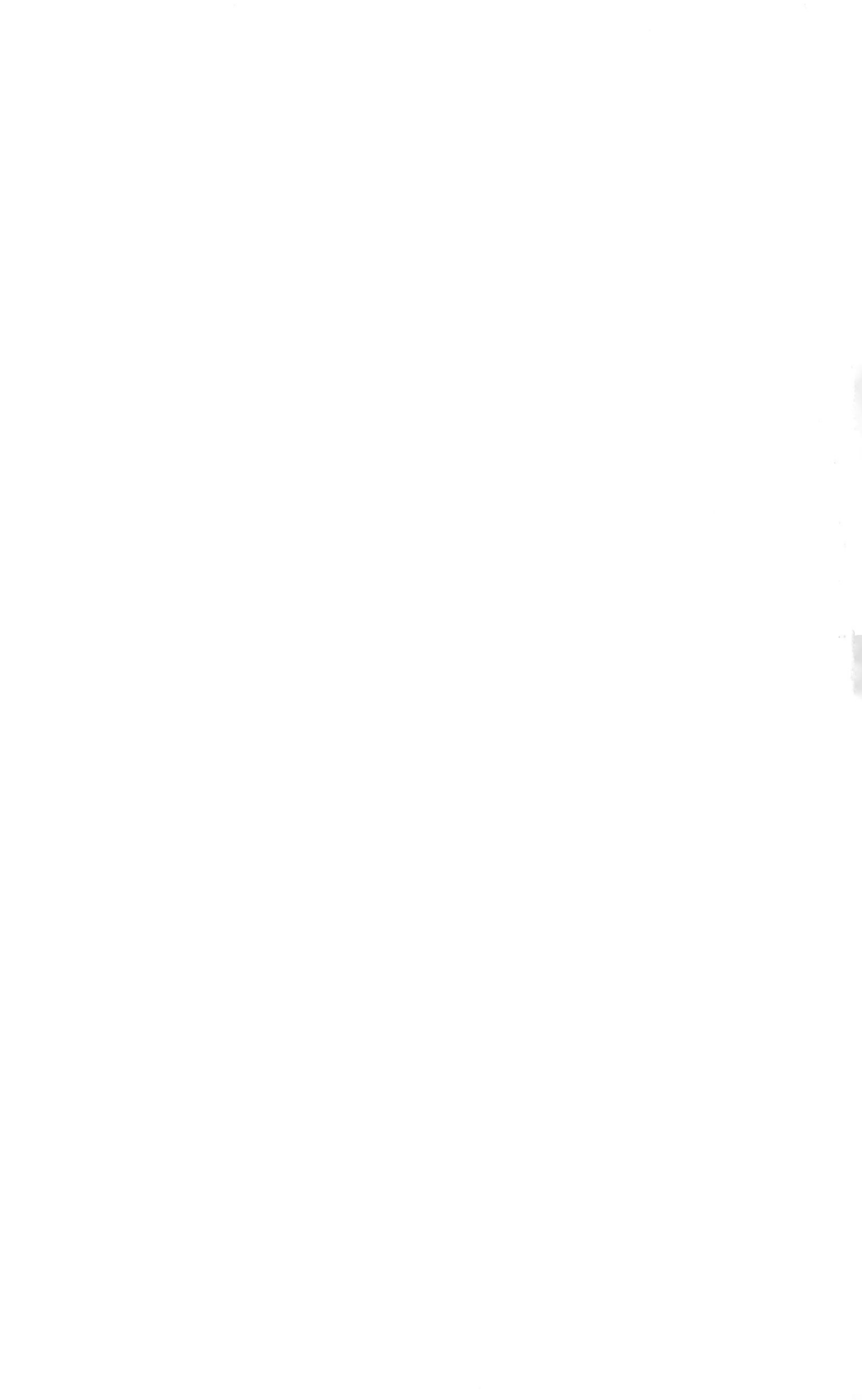

Lightning Source UK Ltd.
Milton Keynes UK
UKHW041416021120
372652UK00010B/2148

9 781988 058436